PRAISE FOR *THE*
EVIDENCE-BASE
CLINICAL NURSES

MW01201286

"Drs. Rivera and Fitzpatrick bring their vast experience and knowledge into a model easily used in nursing practice. It is the goal of all professional practice environments to use evidence effectively and advance new evidence in the care of patients while ensuring cultural health for clinicians. PEACE provides a simple way for clinical nurses to remember and apply the components of evidence-based practice. Thank you for this blueprint for professional practice."

–Sharon Pappas, PhD, RN, NEA-BC, FAAN
Chief Nurse Executive, Emory Healthcare

"Truly an inspired and practical work that creates a framework for evidence-based practice to be a part of our everyday work as nurses. The PEACE model has the power to accelerate clinical inquiry by bedside scientists and all those who support them by improving outcomes and defining our impact as a profession."

–Cole Edmonson, DNP, RN, NEA-BC, FACHE, FAONL, FNAP, FAAN
Chief Experience and Clinical Officer, AMN Healthcare

"Drs. Reynaldo Rivera and Joyce Fitzpatrick have written a down-to-earth, practical, how-to-do-it book on a model that engages the frontline nurse in delivering evidence-driven solutions to questions they ask and problems they identify. The PEACE model is a useful tool for clearly defining questions, accessing and applying the best evidence, and disseminating the results. The time spent exploring the model is well worth the investment."

–David Marshall, JD, DNP, RN, FAAN, FAONL
Senior Vice President and Chief Nursing Executive
Cedars-Sinai

THE PEACE MODEL

Evidence-Based Practice Guide for
CLINICAL NURSES

Reynaldo R. Rivera | DNP, RN, NEA-BC, FAAN
Joyce J. Fitzpatrick | PhD, MBA, RN, FAAN, FNAP

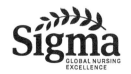

Sigma Theta Tau International Honor Society of Nursing (Sigma) is a nonprofit organization whose mission is developing nurse leaders anywhere to improve healthcare everywhere. Founded in 1922, Sigma has more than 135,000 active members in over 100 countries and territories. Members include practicing nurses, instructors, researchers, policymakers, entrepreneurs, and others. Sigma's more than 540 chapters are located at more than 700 institutions of higher education throughout Armenia, Australia, Botswana, Brazil, Canada, Colombia, England, Eswatini, Ghana, Hong Kong, Ireland, Israel, Jamaica, Japan, Jordan, Kenya, Lebanon, Malawi, Mexico, the Netherlands, Nigeria, Pakistan, Philippines, Portugal, Puerto Rico, Scotland, Singapore, South Africa, South Korea, Sweden, Taiwan, Tanzania, Thailand, the United States, and Wales. Learn more at www.sigmanursing.org.

Sigma Theta Tau International | 550 West North Street, Indianapolis, IN, USA 46202

To request a review copy for course adoption, order additional books, buy in bulk, or purchase for corporate use, contact Sigma Marketplace at 888.654.4968 (US/Canada toll-free), +1.317.687.2256 (International), or solutions@sigmamarketplace.org.

To request author information, or for speaker or other media requests, contact Sigma Marketing at 888.634.7575 (US/Canada toll-free) or +1.317.634.8171 (International).

ISBN: 9781646480104
EPUB ISBN: 9781646480012
PDF ISBN: 9781646480029
MOBI ISBN: 9781646480043

LCCN
2020054402

First Printing, 2021

Publisher: Dustin Sullivan   **Managing Editor:** Carla Hall

Acquisitions Editor: Emily Hatch   **Publications Specialist:** Todd Lothery

Development Editor: Meaghan O'Keeffe   **Project Editor:** Meaghan O'Keeffe

Cover Designer: Michael Tanamachi   **Copy Editor:** Todd Lothery

Interior Design/Page Layout: Michael Tanamachi   **Proofreader:** Gill Editorial Services

Indexer: Larry D. Sweazy

Free Resources

Go to the Sigma Repository for a printable color PEACE model quick reference, a sample chapter, and other useful downloadable materials.

Visit the page at http://hdl.handle.net/10755/21383 or simply scan the QR code below to go directly to the Repository page.

Acknowledgments

The authors wish to recognize the clinical nurses and nurse leaders of NewYork-Presbyterian who participated in the creation of the PEACE model and continued to build the culture of inquiry.

About the Authors

Reynaldo R. Rivera, DNP, RN, NEA-BC, FAAN

Reynaldo R. Rivera is the Director of Nursing Research and Innovation at NewYork-Presbyterian (NYP) and Assistant Professor of Clinical Nursing at Columbia University School of Nursing, both in New York, New York. He is also an Associate Professor of Nursing at Frances Payne Bolton School of Nursing, Case Western Reserve University in Cleveland, Ohio.

In his current role at NYP, he oversees the implementation of evidence-based initiatives, research studies, and practice innovations that will advance nursing science and improve patient outcomes/care. Rivera's research and contributions focus on nurse engagement and practice innovations including nurse residency program, academic-practice collaboration initiatives, mentoring, narrative nursing, appreciative inquiry, use of liberating structures, and enhancing professional governance.

Rivera served as a board member of the American Organization for Nursing Leadership, Advisory Board of the Duke-Johnson & Johnson Nurse Leadership Program, President of the American Association of Critical Care Nurses (AACN) New York City Chapter, and President of the Philippine Nurses Association of America.

He is a board member of the American Association for Men in Nursing (AAMN) Foundation as well as an advisory board of the Rockefeller University, Heilbrunn Family for Research Nursing. He has received many prestigious awards, such as the Teachers College, Columbia University Outstanding Alumni Award, AACN Flame of Excellence Award, and the AAMN Lee Cohen Award. He is a fellow of the American Academy of Nursing and of the Academy's Selection Committee.

Rivera received his BSN from University of the East Ramon Magsaysay Memorial Medical Center in the Philippines; MA in assessment and measurement psychology from Ateneo de Manila University, Philippines; MA and EdM in nursing executive role from Teachers College, Columbia University, New York; Post Masters in advanced nursing practice from New York University, New York; and Doctor of Nursing Practice from Frances Payne Bolton School of Nursing, Case Western Reserve University in Ohio.

Joyce J. Fitzpatrick, PhD, MBA, RN, FAAN, FNAP

Joyce J. Fitzpatrick is the Inaugural Director of the Marian K. Shaughnessy Nurse Leadership Academy and Elizabeth Brooks Ford Professor of Nursing, Frances Payne Bolton School of Nursing, Case Western Reserve University (CWRU) in Cleveland, Ohio, where she was Dean from 1982 through 1997. Fitzpatrick is widely published in nursing and healthcare literature with over 400 publications, including more than 80 books. She served as coeditor of the *Annual Review of Nursing Research* series, Volumes 1–26. She is editor of the classic *Encyclopedia of Nursing Research*, now in its 4th edition, and coeditor of the *Encyclopedia of Nursing Education*. Currently she edits the journals *Applied Nursing Research* and *Archives in Psychiatric Nursing*.

From 1997–1999 she served as President of the American Academy of Nursing (AAN); she currently serves as Vice-Chair of the American Nurses Foundation. She has received numerous honors and awards; she was elected a Fellow in the American Academy of Nursing in 1981, Fellow in the National Academies of Practice in 1996, and an Honorary Fellow of the American Academy of Nurse Practitioners in 2018. She received the *American Journal of Nursing* Book of the Year Award 20 times. In 2014 Fitzpatrick was inducted into the STTI Research Hall of Fame. In 2016 she was named a Living Legend by AAN, and in 2018 she received the prestigious ANA Jessie M. Scott Award that recognizes leadership in demonstrating the interdependence between nursing education, practice, and research. In June 2019 she was awarded the International Council of Nurses and Florence Nightingale Foundation International Achievement Award, recognizing her contribution to advancing international nursing education through research, innovative conceptual models, and theory development.

She earned a BSN (Georgetown University), an MS in psychiatric-mental health nursing (The Ohio State University), a PhD in nursing (New York University), and an MBA (CWRU). In 1990, Fitzpatrick received an honorary doctorate, Doctor of Humane Letters, from Georgetown University. In 2011 she received an honorary doctorate, Doctor of Humane Letters, from the Frontier University of Nursing.

Contributing Authors

Eileen Carter, PhD, RN

Eileen Carter is an Assistant Professor at Columbia University School of Nursing and Nurse Researcher, NewYork-Presbyterian Hospital, both in New York, New York.

Carter is an emergency department nurse by background and passionate about advancing nurses' contributions to improved patient safety and outcomes. She has received national grant funding to pursue her research interests regarding healthcare-associated infection prevention and antibiotic resistance. Upon completing her PhD in 2014, she was the first to enter a novel jointly appointed research role spanning Columbia University School of Nursing and NewYork-Presbyterian Hospital, in which a portion of her total effort is dedicated to facilitating clinical scholarship among nurses in practice settings.

Kenrick D. Cato, PhD, RN, CPHIMS, FAAN

Kenrick D. Cato is a Nurse Researcher/Assistant Professor for NewYork-Presbyterian Hospital and Columbia University School of Nursing, respectively. Cato has a varied background. He worked at NewYork-Presbyterian Health system as a surgical and medical oncology clinical nurse and as an analyst in the information technology department, working on projects to improve patient safety through the use of clinical decision support (CDS). In the analyst position, he focused on projects to improve patient safety through the optimization of the hospital's electronic systems. Cato's program of research focuses on the mining of electronic patient data to support clinical decision-making. His previous work includes National Institute of Health-funded research in health communication via mobile health platforms, shared decision-making in primary care settings, and data mining of electronic patient records. His current projects include automated data mining of electronic patient records to discover patient characters that are often missed and the development of predictive models for inpatient clinical deterioration.

Bevin Cohen, PhD, MS, MPH, RN

Bevin Cohen is the Director of Research and Evidence-Based Practice at Mount Sinai Hospital, New York, New York. Cohen received her PhD and MPH in epidemiology and MS in nursing from Columbia University and her BA in public health from the University of Vermont. Her previous research roles include appointments as Associate Research Scientist and Program Director at Columbia University School of Nursing and Nurse Scientist at Memorial Sloan Kettering Cancer Center.

Laarni C. Florencio, MSN, RN, CNL

Laarni C. Florencio is the Program Director for Continuing Education at NewYork-Presbyterian (NYP). She oversees continuing nursing education events for all 11 NYP facilities and collaborates with Weill Cornell Medical College and Columbia Medical schools, both Ivy League-recognized Medical Schools in New York for Nursing and Interprofessional Continuing Education courses. She earned her master's degree in nursing from Florida Atlantic University and her postgraduate certificate degree in evidence-based practice from the University of Maryland School of Nursing. She currently maintains her certification as a Clinical Nurse Leader through the American Association of Colleges of Nursing (AACN) and is enrolled in the Doctor of Nursing Practice degree program at Frances Payne Bolton School of Nursing, Case Western Reserve University.

Michele P. Holskey, DNP, RN, NEA-BC

Michele Price Holskey is an Assistant Professor in the Nursing Program at Coastal Carolina University and Magnet Consultant, NewYork-Presbyterian Hospital, in New York, New York. In addition to her role as a medical-surgical and diabetes Clinical Nurse Specialist, Holskey is an experienced nurse leader and former Chief Nurse Executive who has spent a significant portion of her career facilitating and writing about the contributions of professional nurses to patients, organizations, professions, and communities. She assists organizations on their journey to achieve recognition for nursing excellence. Holskey is a Fundamentals of Magnet® certificate holder and passionate educator for nursing leadership, health policy, nursing informatics and data management, nursing research, and population health. Her current projects include the integration of liberating structures for optimizing student and nurse engagement. She received her BSN and MSN degrees from the University of Virginia and her Doctor of Nursing Practice degree from Case Western Reserve University Frances Payne Bolton School of Nursing.

Kristine M. Kulage, MA, MPH

Kristine M. Kulage is the Director of Research and Scholarly Development at Columbia University School of Nursing, New York, New York. She has been employed in research administration for nearly 25 years, with 17 years at Columbia Nursing, and currently focuses on increasing the research and scholarly capacity of nursing faculty members. Originally obtaining a BA and MA in English/composition, she started her academic career teaching college writing classes and has brought those skills full circle by leading efforts aimed at improving scholarly writing and dissemination. In 2014, she earned an MPH in health policy and management, enabling her to participate more substantially in the grant writing efforts of research faculty members she supports. She leads numerous writing-focused workshops throughout the year, including a peer-reviewed manuscript writing workshop, an annual workshop for PhD students focused on writing grant applications to support their dissertation work, and an annual workshop for postdoctoral trainees focused on writing career development awards. In addition to serving as an ad hoc reviewer for professional journals, she has been the managing editor of the *Journal of Doctoral Nursing Practice* since 2015. She has presented orally and via posters at numerous conferences and has 14 professional articles in PubMed.

Keith C. Mages, PhD, MLS, MSN, RN, AHIP

Keith C. Mages is the Norton M. Luger, MD Clinical Medical Librarian at the Samuel J. Wood Library of Weill Cornell Medicine (WCM). In this role, he provides research and evidence-based practice support to practicing nurses, physicians, medical fellows, residents, and students. Mages also provides caregiver and consumer health education at the point of care, in NewYork-Presbyterian Hospital/Weill Cornell (NYP/WC). He is a member of the Medical Library Association (MLA) and a senior member of the Academy of Health Information Professionals. He has been awarded the Presidential Award from the MLA Board of Directors for his work on the Educational Steering Committee, the coordinating body for MLA educational initiatives. Mages serves on the NYP/WC Ethics Committee, as an Ethics Faculty Tutor at WCM, and as an Adjunct Faculty member of New York University's Rory Meyers College of Nursing. His publication and funding record reflect his research interests in health literacy, consumer health education, and the history of health sciences. Mages received his BS in nursing and MLS in library and information science from the University at Buffalo – SUNY, an MSN in advanced practice child and adolescent psychiatric nursing from Yale University, as well as a PhD in the history of nursing from the University of Pennsylvania.

Kevin D. Masick, PhD

Kevin D. Masick is a principal consultant for Moving Targets Consulting and adjunct faculty at Hofstra University. He has more than 15 years in healthcare leading analytics, education, and research as well as many years teaching undergraduate and graduate research methodology and statistics. He has been an author of Research Methods: Designing and Conducting Research with a Real-World Focus and Storytelling with Data in Healthcare. Masick completed his PhD in Applied Organizational Psychology and his master of arts degree in Industrial and Organizational Psychology from Hofstra University, New York, New York. He completed his bachelor of arts in psychology from State University of New York in Albany, New York.

Allison A. Norful, PhD, RN, ANP-BC

Allison Norful is an Assistant Professor, Columbia University School of Nursing and Nurse Researcher, NewYork-Presbyterian Hospital, New York, New York. Norful has more than two decades of clinical, administrative, and research experience. She completed her PhD in nursing from Columbia University School of Nursing, her master of science in nursing at New York University, New York, New York, and her bachelors of science in nursing at LaSalle University. She completed her post-doctoral fellowship in medicine and formal training in health services research and comparative effectiveness studies at Columbia University, New York, New York.

Jessica O'Brien Gufarotti, MS, RN, AGCNS-BC, PCCN

Jessica O'Brien Gufarotti is a Clinical Nurse Specialist (CNS) at NewYork-Presbyterian Lower Manhattan Hospital. As a CNS, O'Brien Gufarotti focuses on three domains: the patient and family, the nurse, and the system. Furthermore, she provides support to nurses caring for patients at the bedside, ensures the use of best practices and evidence-based care, and drives practice change throughout the organization to help safeguard optimal patient and organizational outcomes. O'Brien Gufarotti is currently involved in multiple projects to help advance nursing practice and improve patient outcomes. She received her Master of Science from the Hunter-Bellevue School of Nursing in 2017 and her bachelor in nursing at SUNY Plattsburgh in 2010.

Mary Rose Papciak, MPA, BSN, RN, NEA-BC

Mary Rose Papciak earned her master's degree in public administration from New York University and maintains her certification as Nurse Executive Advanced through the American Nurses Credentialing Center (ANCC). Papciak is the Program Director for Professional Nursing Practice Innovation at NewYork-Presbyterian Hospital (NYPH). She is responsible for the transition to practice program of new graduate nurses for seven sites across New York City. She also collaborates with Nursing Leadership teams throughout the enterprise to facilitate the Mentorship Program and supports innovative practices to advance the profession of nursing. Papciak is thankful to have the opportunity to give back to new nurses, inspire them, and watch them grow. In her position, she can support and educate nurses to improve bedside care. She has the ability to promote health and well-being as a nurse by demonstrating care for those who are caring for others. Her passions include staff engagement and "inspiring it forward" to elevate the nursing profession. As a believer in the difference nurses make, Papciak remains committed to the success of new graduate nurses, not only at NYP, but throughout our nation. She is an avid runner and Pilates enthusiast.

Warly Remegio, DNP, MS, RN-BC, CCRN-CSC

Warly Remegio is the Program Director of Nursing Professional Development at NewYork-Presbyterian/Lower Manhattan Hospital. In his role, he leads a team of educators and oversees all the education and nursing professional development activities throughout the organization. Using his leadership and nursing professional development expertise for over 10 years, he facilitates the development and implementation of programs and initiatives that foster culture of inquiry. Prior to this appointment, Remegio assumed a dual role as Professional Development Manager and Critical Care Education Specialist in the Center for Professional Practice Excellence at Holy Name Medical Center (HNMC), Teaneck, New Jersey. At HNMC, he cultivated a culture of inquiry by leading the Generating New Knowledge Council. He advanced nursing practice by championing evidence-based practice, research, and performance improvement projects within the organization. Remegio completed his Doctor of Nursing Practice degree at Frances Payne Bolton School of Nursing at Case Western Reserve University (2020) and his Master of Science, concentration on Healthcare Management and Nurse Executive Program (2008) and Post Masters Certificate-Adult Nurse Practitioner (2015) at Long Island University, Brooklyn, New York, New York.

Alexandra N. Shelley, MS, RN-BC, FNP-BC

Alexandra Shelley is the Magnet Program Director and was previously a Clinical Program Coordinator at NewYork-Presbyterian Lower Manhattan Hospital, New York, New York. Shelley has had many years of experience in implementing and leading evidence-based change projects. She has served as the chair of her organization's EBP and Research Committee and now serves on the committee as an EBP Mentor. As a clinical nurse, Shelley was instrumental in the creation and dissemination of the PEACE model. Alexa received her master of science in nursing, Family Nurse Practitioner program from Columbia University in 2017 and her Bachelor of Science in nursing from University of Pennsylvania with Magna Cum Laude in 2009.

Carolyn Sun, PhD, RN, ANP-BC

Carolyn Sun is an Assistant Professor at Hunter-Bellevue School of Nursing, Hunter College, New York, New York. She also holds an appointment at Columbia University School of Nursing, Columbia University, New York, New York, and consults as a Nurse Researcher for NewYork-Presbyterian Hospital in New York, New York. She was previously employed with a joint appointment as an Associate Research Scientist, Columbia University School of Nursing, Columbia University, New York, New York, and a Nurse Researcher, NewYork-Presbyterian. Sun did her post-doctoral studies in Global Health at Columbia University School of Nursing,

Columbia University, and completed her PhD in Nursing at Columbia University School of Nursing, Columbia University. Sun completed her masters of science in nursing, Adult Nurse Practitioner, at New York University, New York, New York. She completed her undergraduate Nursing Degree at Bellevue College in Bellevue, Washington, and her bachelor of art degree in art with a minor in biology from Seattle Pacific University, in Seattle, Washington.

Haofei Wang, DNP, RN, NEA-BC

Haofei Wang is a nurse leader with over 20 years of experience in nursing practice and quality. She is Director of Professional Nursing Practice at NewYork-Presbyterian responsible for the development and maintenance of programs within Nursing that support and evaluate nursing practice, while meeting the requirements of the Joint Commission, NYS Department of Health, and professional practice standards. Wang held her previous position as the Director of Nursing Practice and Quality at the Regional Hospital Network at NewYork-Presbyterian. As part of her responsibilities, Wang led the nursing practice, quality, and education standardization across the regional hospitals as well as the full integration of Lawrence Hospital as the seventh NYPH campus. She supported the implementation of the Professional Governance structures at NYP/Brooklyn Methodist, NYP/Queens, and Gracie Square Hospital. Wang is a member of the Sigma Theta Tau International Honor Society of Nursing and the American Organization of Nurse Executives and has presented locally and internationally. She obtained her Doctor of Nursing Practice from George Washington University in 2017, her master of science in nursing from the University of Phoenix in 2008, and her bachelor of science in nursing from Georgetown University in 1998.

Table of Contents

Foreword

There is no question that the best prepared nurses must be available to provide patient and family-centered nursing care. Nurses are the backbone of all healthcare systems, often the heart and soul, ever present, providing 24-hour care. Without well-prepared nurses, our healthcare systems would not be as effective in meeting the needs of the many individuals, families, and communities we serve.

At NewYork-Presbyterian (NYP), nurses are key in improving the quality of patient and family-centered care. We also know that without the structure of the PEACE model to prepare all new and continuing nurses, we would not have the quality outcomes that have led to Magnet® designation for several of our hospitals. Our model for implementing evidence-based practice (EBP) and research is exemplary. From the EBP Deep-Dive sessions that are implemented with clinical nurses and the Nurse Residency Program that has been highly successful with new graduates, we believe that NYP is poised to continue to deliver the best healthcare and improve patient care outcomes.

Without question, part of the success of our endeavors has been our partnerships with academic nursing institutions. Our colleagues in academic research and scholarship have continued to share their expertise, just as our clinical nurses have shared their expertise in patient and family-centered care delivery. Academic-practice partnerships provide models for future success. We have successful models in place that can be adapted within other hospitals, large and small. Many examples included in this book showcase the academic-practice collaborations that we have initiated and continue to develop.

Throughout NYP we have created effective quality structures and implemented process improvements that have led to highly desirable patient care outcomes. We believe that these can be replicated in other institutions. The uniqueness of the PEACE model of evidence-based practice is its appeal to the clinical nurses who are providing care at the bedside. Our new and experienced nurses acclaim the value of the PEACE model for guiding their practice and research. It is a mnemonic that is easy to remember, particularly given today's times of social turmoil. Clinical nurses gravitate toward an understanding of the value of peace in their everyday work, with the patient who is experiencing a health crisis to assistance with family members who are bewildered about the complexity of the healthcare delivery system to the population health issues that abound in our communities and demand evidence-based solutions to care delivery.

Nurses are obligated to fulfill their compact with society, to deliver on the care promises that are an inherent part of their professional licensure. At NYP, we believe we have an obligation to lead the way to better care for each patient and their family members and for our communities and our broader societies. We also believe that the PEACE model will drive quality care toward our end goal: excellence in care for all.

Wilhelmina (Willie) M. Manzano
MA, RN, NEA- BC, FAAN
Senior Vice President
Chief Nursing Executive
& Chief Quality Officer
NewYork-Presbyterian, New York, New York

Introduction

–Reynaldo R. Rivera, DNP, RN, NEA-BC, FAAN
–Joyce J. Fitzpatrick, PhD, MBA, RN, FAAN, FNAP

"Let whoever is in charge keep this simple question in her head (not, how can I always do this right thing myself) how can I provide for this right thing to be always done."

–Florence Nightingale

Nurses are in charge of the patients and their families throughout the hospital and health system experience. They assist patients through illness to achieve higher levels of health. They coordinate the care throughout the patients' experiences with the healthcare system. Nurses are the leaders of patient care at the bedside and beyond. It is important that as clinical leaders, nurses have the most accurate, most up-to-date, and evidence-based information available so that they can always do the right thing. The PEACE model develops clinical nurses as leaders in care of both patients and their families. Clinical nurses, those at the point of care, have embraced this model for guiding their practice. The PEACE model helps clinical nurses solve challenging problems through a rigorous evidence-based practice process—from problem identification to evaluation and dissemination.

The crux of the PEACE model is the mnemonic that simplifies the evidence-based practice (EBP) process for clinical nurses. The PEACE model is used across NewYork-Presbyterian (NYP), one of the nation's most comprehensive academic healthcare delivery systems. NYP is composed of 10 hospitals in New York and employs more than 11,000 nurses across the enterprise.

One striking advantage of the model is that it emerged from the work of clinical nurses who were struggling to find a way to remember and apply the components of other EBP models. Clinical nurses have indicated that the components of the PEACE model make the model memorable and useful (see Figure I.1):

P for problem identification

E for evidence review

A for appraising the evidence

C for changing practice or conducting research

E for evaluating and disseminating the findings

PEACE Model

PROBLEM IDENTIFICATION

Formulate the clinical question (**PICO**):

P | Patient Population
I | Intervention
C | Comparison of Intervention
O | Outcome

EVIDENCE REVIEW

Review evidence relevant to your clinical question by searching databases.

APPRAISE EVIDENCE

Appraise the evidence that appears highest in the hierarchy of scientific evidence for its quality and applicability to practice.

CHANGE PRACTICE OR CONDUCT RESEARCH

If evidence is sufficient, embark on improvement project to address practice change.
If evidence is insufficient to warrant practice change, conduct research.

EVALUATE AND DISSEMINATE FINDINGS

Evaluate the impact of the implemented practice change and research results.
Disseminate findings through publication, oral, and poster presentations.

Figure I.1 | NYP PEACE model.

The last stage of the PEACE model is particularly important to advancing nursing practice across institutions. We have found that unless the model results are disseminated through scholarly presentations and publications, the clinical challenges continue to be present across sites and institutions. We emphasize this phase and conduct publication workshops to help clinical nurses shape the dissemination of their EBP work. Nurses' active participation in EBP and research is critical to improving the care we provide to patients and furthering nursing science. It is important to note that the design of the PEACE model intentionally linked EBP, quality improvement (QI), and research.

Uniqueness of PEACE Model

The mnemonic PEACE promotes understanding and application by clinical nurses, providing a way to easily remember the EBP component stages. The uniqueness of the PEACE model is its simplicity. This relevance leads to continued application in day-to-day nursing practice. As we strive for peace at many levels of our lives and work, the mnemonic is easy to remember. The PEACE model may be adapted to any setting where nurses practice.

Goals of the Book

After reading this book, you will have the opportunities to:

- Differentiate between EBP, research, and quality improvement.
- Discuss the PEACE model process from problem identification to dissemination of findings.
- Identify resources to support nurses in EBP, quality improvement, and conducting research.

Organization of the Book

The chapters are organized using the five-step EBP process, including chapters addressing differentiating research, EBP, QI, resources, and practice exemplars.

Chapter 1: This chapter provides defining principles, similarities and differences in EBP, QI, and research when pursuing scholarly EBP projects, QI activities, and research studies.

Chapter 2: This chapter centers on the first step of the PEACE model, which uses a specialized framework known as PICO (Population, Intervention, Comparison Intervention, and Outcome) to formulate a meaningful clinical question that would facilitate an effective search for existing literature.

Chapter 3: The second step of the PEACE model is evidence review, which consists of a literature review of the most current research findings utilizing available databases. Learners are introduced to the nuts and bolts of literature searching—use of Boolean operators, controlled vocabulary, keywords, truncation, and limits and management of evidence retrieved.

Chapter 4: The third step of the PEACE model is to appraise the evidence. Appraising evidence guides nurses to evaluate the levels and quality of the evidence and determine whether there is sufficient evidence to initiate a practice change or embark on an additional research study.

Chapter 5: The fourth step of the PEACE model is either to change practice or to conduct research—if evidence is sufficient, then change practice. This chapter provides steps in planning and implementing EBP change and strategies to sustain practice changes.

Chapter 6: If you determine that there is insufficient evidence to warrant practice change or a gap in knowledge, then the next logical step is to conduct research. This chapter focuses on developing a research plan that is grounded or well thought out, designing sound research methods that are clear of ethical quandaries.

Chapter 7: The fifth step of the PEACE model is to evaluate and disseminate findings. This chapter centers on the evaluation of implemented practice change and research results. It focuses on the importance of planning projects, especially on outcome measures.

Chapter 8: This chapter focuses on the importance of disseminating findings through publication, oral, and poster presentations.

Chapter 9: This chapter describes NYP's resources that you may adapt in your institutions to build the culture of inquiry.

Chapter 10: This chapter provides exemplars of EBP and research that utilize the PEACE model.

Utilization of the PEACE Model

The PEACE model is an integral component of NYP's Nurse Residency Program, which supports new graduate nurses' transition from advanced beginners to competent nurses. All EBP projects completed by new graduate nurse residents utilized the PEACE model. NYP's Nurse Residency Program has received accreditation with distinction from the American Nurses Credentialing Center, a recognition for excellence in transitioning nurses to new practice settings. The PEACE model may be adopted by the nurse residency program as you build your culture of inquiry in your institutions.

We also provided classes on EBP/Research Deep Dive, where nurses receive hands-on guidance on how to proceed with a research idea or question utilizing the NYP PEACE model. This book will be a resource for our nurses who are interested in knowing a simple, concise, and easy-to-use PEACE model.

Educational Relevance

Based on its relevance to clinical nurses, the PEACE model is particularly suited to RN to BSN students as well as students in prelicensure BSN programs. This book may be used in several clinical courses to illustrate the work that practicing nurses initiate and can be used in specific EBP courses. At the graduate education level, the book may be used as a required text or supplementary reference for both EBP and research courses, as there are several examples that address the components relevant to each of the EBP and research processes. The nurses who have used the model in their clinical work at NYP have indicated that it also is useful in their academic pursuits. In addition to the applications within formal academic programs, we have found the PEACE model relevant to continuing education programs across a wide range of clinical specialties.

We hope that nurses will find this book a road map from delineating the steps of how to formulate and address a clinical question to the dissemination of findings. We believe that nurses' integration of evidence at the bedside and conduct of research are foundational to advancing nursing science, improving the care we provide to patients, and achieving optimal patient outcomes.

PEACE MODEL

P | **PROBLEM IDENTIFICATION**
Formulate the clinical question (**PICO**):
- **P** | Patient Population
- **I** | Intervention
- **C** | Comparison of Intervention
- **O** | Outcome

E | **EVIDENCE REVIEW**
Review evidence relevant to your clinical question by searching databases.

A | **APPRAISE EVIDENCE**
Appraise the evidence that appears highest in the hierarchy of scientific evidence for its quality and applicability to practice.

C | **CHANGE PRACTICE OR CONDUCT RESEARCH**
If evidence is sufficient, embark on improvement project to address practice change.
If evidence is insufficient to warrant practice change, conduct research.

E | **EVALUATE AND DISSEMINATE FINDINGS**
Evaluate the impact of the implemented practice change and research results.
Disseminate findings through publication, oral, and poster presentations.

1

EVIDENCE-BASED PRACTICE, RESEARCH, AND QUALITY IMPROVEMENT

—Eileen Carter, PhD, RN

KEYWORDS | PHRASES

clinical scholarship, evidence-based practice, quality improvement, research, institutional review board

---

CHAPTER OBJECTIVES

After studying this chapter, learners will be able to:

1. Describe the defining principles of evidence-based practice, quality improvement, and research.
2. Recognize instances in which evidence-based practice, quality improvement, and research overlap.
3. Describe the defining attributes of research.

Introduction

Clinical nurses are increasingly leading projects to improve patient care. Professional nursing and medical bodies alike recognize the uniquely important role nurses have in identifying and addressing clinical improvement opportunities and encourage nurses to be actively engaged in such areas. The National Academy of Medicine (formerly called the Institute of Medicine) and the American Association of Colleges of Nursing specify evidence-based practice and quality improvement approaches as core competencies for nurses (American Association of Colleges of Nursing, 2008; Institute of Medicine [US] Committee on the Health Professions Education Summit et al., 2003). Similarly, the American Nurses Credentialing Center, which recognizes hospitals reaching pinnacle levels of nursing excellence, includes nurses' conduct of research, evidence-based practice, and quality improvement as standards for Magnet® designation.

This chapter provides practical tips for clinical nurses to help them determine the types of activities necessary to solve clinical problems. Also identified are instances in which activities may become blurred. Importantly, in the chapter there is emphasis on the importance of following established frameworks and models to guide scholarly work.

The PEACE Model: A Framework for Evidence-Based Practice

While evidence-based practice, quality improvement, and research exist along the continuum of clinical scholarship (Carter et al., 2017), each has its own unique set of principles and procedures that should be followed. Thus, clinical nurses are challenged with identifying the type of activity they wish to embark upon to ensure that the activity is methodologically sound and meets institutional, local, and federal requirements (in the case of research). Numerous authors describe differences in evidence-based practice, quality improvement, and research (Baker et al., 2014; Carter et al., 2017; Fitzpatrick, 2016; Shirey et al., 2011). Yet, the categorization of these activities remains a source of confusion, especially in real-world clinical settings, where activities may overlap. For instance, these activities may be a combination of quality improvement and research or evolve over time and begin as an evidence-based practice project and add dimensions that involve a research study.

Evidence-based practice (EBP) is the active integration of best research evidence, clinician expertise, and patient preferences in the care of patients (Sackett et al., 1996). The EBP movement began in the 1990s, after studies showed substantial gaps between the treatments that we know work and the treatments given to patients. Hand hygiene among healthcare workers is an example of one such gap. Hand hygiene is considered the most effective means to prevent infection, and for decades, the Centers for Disease Control and Prevention and the World Health Organization have published hand hygiene guidelines to effectively aid in the prevention of infections (Boyce & Pittet, 2002; Pittet et al., 2009). Despite guidelines specifying that healthcare workers perform hand hygiene before and after patient contact to prevent infections, average hand hygiene compliance remains suboptimal (Erasmus et al., 2010; Lambe et al., 2019). Thus, there remains a large chasm between the care that we know is in the best interest of patients and the care that is given to patients, and this underscores the need for nurses' active engagement in EBP.

In general, EBP is characterized by nurses' performance of five steps (Stevens, 2013):

1) Identify a clinical issue
2) Review research evidence pertaining to the clinical issue
3) Appraise the evidence for quality
4) Incorporate evidence into patient care (as applicable) and in conjunction with patient preferences and nursing expertise
5) Evaluate the impact of activities on patient care. Numerous evidence-based models exist to guide nurses in these five steps.

The PEACE model (described in the introduction and explored in the subsequent chapters of this book) is NewYork-Presbyterian's evidence-based framework. This PEACE model was developed by and for nurses at NewYork-Presbyterian to guide evidence-based decision-making (Tahan et al., 2016).

Real-World Example of EBP

Remy is an emergency department (ED) nurse who recently began working at an ED closer to home. Remy notices that decisions to insert urinary catheters differ at his new institution. For instance, in his new institution, urinary catheters are routinely used among patients with incontinence, whereas this was not the case in his previous work setting. Remy knows that patients who receive urinary catheters are at risk for catheter-associated urinary tract infections (CAUTI) and wants to ensure that only patients with a medically appropriate reason for a urinary catheter receive a urinary catheter.

This real-world example provides a typical starting point to launching an EBP project. Here, a nurse identifies a clinical question ("What is the medical appropriateness criteria for urinary catheters?") after observing variation in the performance of practices (decisions to insert urinary catheters) and recognizing the implications of care (use of urinary catheters) on patient outcomes (CAUTI). In this scenario, nurses would follow the five-step evidence-based nursing process in formulating a clinical question, reviewing pertinent literature, appraising pertinent literature for its quality and applicability, integrating the literature in the care of patients, and evaluating the impact of activities on patient outcomes. At times, the evidence-based nursing process is not always used or correctly followed. For instance, steps of the evidence-based nursing process may be skipped or followed out of sequence, which can result in adverse consequences for patients and staff. The following theoretical example demonstrates such a scenario.

CASE STUDY:

Importance of Following the Five-Step Evidence-Based Nursing Process

Scenario

Nurse Amber is a clinical nurse in an adult medical-surgical unit who leads her Unit Practice Committee. Falls are a problem on the unit. Nurse Amber and members of the Unit Practice Committee are eager to embark on an EBP project to prevent falls. Through discussion, the committee members decide the best way to prevent falls on their unit is to ensure that all patients receive bed alarms.

The committee members implement the project by placing all patients on bed alarms. Remember, this is a theoretical example! The widespread use of bed alarms leads to the constant sounding of alarms, causes frustration among patients, and intensifies alarm fatigue among staff. As a result, bed alarms are ignored rather than addressed, which perpetuates patient harm.

Discussion

An intervention (widespread use of bed alarms on all patients) that is not supported by current evidence was implemented and resulted in adverse consequences for patients and staff.

In this example, committee members skipped three steps that are critical to evidence-based decision-making: development of a clinical question and the review and appraisal of relevant research evidence.

Clinical Implications

Nurses are leading unit-based projects that have substantial bearing on patient care and outcomes. When conducting EBP, clinical nurses should sequentially follow the five-step evidence-based nursing process to ensure that changes in practice are rooted in high-quality evidence.

Quality Improvement

Quality improvement includes data-driven approaches that aim to improve care locally. Numerous quality improvement approaches and strategies exist—the Model for Improvement, Plan Do Study Act (PDSA) cycles (Agency for Healthcare Research and Quality, 2013), Six Sigma, Lean, and so on—to guide the conduct of quality improvement activities. A real-world example of nurses' use of PDSA to guide a quality improvement activity is provided in the next section.

Real-World Example of Quality Improvement

Nurse Adriana works as a clinical nurse in a medical-surgical unit of an adult hospital. Her hospital recently implemented Fall Tailored Interventions for Patient Safety (TIPS) after the program was found to significantly reduce falls in the inpatient setting (Dykes et al., 2010). Fall TIPS is characterized by healthcare workers' active engagement and partnership with patients throughout the three-step fall prevention plan: 1) identifying risk factors for falls using a valid and reliable assessment tool; 2) developing fall prevention plans that are evidence-based, tailored to individual patients, and informed by decision support; and 3) consistently implementing individual fall prevention plans over time.

Adriana believes the active engagement of patients in falls is critical to falls prevention and is confident that Fall TIPS will help to prevent falls on her unit. During a recent huddle, however, Adriana's nurse manager reports that the incidence of falls has substantially increased on their unit, and root cause analyses show that patients are not being adequately engaged in falls prevention. The manager asks for volunteers to embark on a falls prevention initiative, with a principal focus on improved patient engagement.

Adriana volunteers to lead the initiative and is delighted that several of her peers express interest in participating. She recommends that the group uses the PDSA framework, as it will standardize their process and ensure a sensible approach to their efforts, in which process and outcomes are monitored and evaluated. Guided by PDSA, the group decides to use publicly available tools (http://www.falltips.org/) to educate staff on effective patient engagement strategies in falls prevention (plan); carry out the education and collect relevant audit data to assess patient engagement procedures (do); evaluate the impact of the intervention on the incidence of patient falls (study); and modify the approach as necessary (act).

While existing quality improvement approaches and strategies should guide quality improvement frameworks, individuals may intentionally or unintentionally forgo these resources due to a lack of awareness of existing resources or a belief that existing resources are no better than intuition alone. Yet, when these valuable resources are overlooked, individuals may spend considerable time and energy developing processes and strategies to guide projects. The prudent approach is for individuals to identify an appropriate framework and accompanying strategies at the outset of the project and adapt these according to project needs.

Research

Research is systematic inquiry that aims to generate or refine existing knowledge (Grady, 2018). While the conduct of research may be unfamiliar to some practicing nurses, studies show that clinical nurses are increasingly serving as the principal investigator or coinvestigator on their clinical units (Cato et al., 2019). Indeed, nurses are uniquely positioned to identify critical gaps and opportunities in patient care that are ripe for research given their routine patient care responsibilities and continual presence at the patient's bedside (Powell, 2015). When nurses question whether the activity they wish to conduct is research, two questions should be asked at a minimum. If the activity is designed to contribute to generalizable knowledge and if the activity will be conducted using information gained from humans, the activity meets the federal definition of research activities, and institutional review board (IRB) approval is needed. These questions are included in Table 1.1.

Table 1.1 | Determining Whether Activity Is Research

Research Criteria	Yes	No
1. Is the activity designed to contribute to generalizable knowledge?		
2. Will the activity be conducted using information gathered from humans? (e.g., conducting a medical chart review of patients, surveying patients, staff, etc.)		

*If the answer to *both* questions is yes, the activity is research, and IRB approval is needed.

Research activities must meet federal and local regulations as well as institutional policies and procedures (Slutsman & Nieman, 2018). The IRB is an independent ethics committee that ensures research studies meet such requirements and are conducted in accordance with the ethical principles that guide clinical research (Grady, 2018). Importantly, IRB approval is needed for research activities to begin. Ethical concepts integral to the conduct of research include 1) *respect for persons*, meaning that individuals are autonomous in deciding to participate or not to participate in research; 2) *beneficence*, meaning that harms to research participants are minimized while benefits to research participants are maximized; and 3) *justice*, meaning fair distribution in the selection of research participants (Grady, 2018). A real-world example of research principles in action follows.

Real-World Example of Ethical Principles in Nursing Research

Nurses Ingrid and Estria are interested in conducting interviews and focus groups with nurses and prescribers to explore their experiences and attitudes toward nurses' involvement in antibiotic stewardship (i.e., efforts to improve the appropriate route, dose, duration, and selection of antibiotics). They recognize they are conducting research, as they intend to develop knowledge that is generalizable beyond their settings of work.

Before they embark on their study, they submit a protocol describing their research plans to their institution's IRB and await IRB approval. In the research protocol, Ingrid and Estria carefully describe how they will conduct their study in accordance with the ethical principles that guide research. In particular, they delineate informed consent procedures and specify that potential research participants will be provided information about the study orally and in writing. Such information will include the purpose of the study, conditions of participation, risks of and benefits to participation, and that study participation is completely voluntary (*respect for persons*). Similarly, in the protocol, Ingrid and Estria specify how harms to research participants will be minimized and benefits maximized. In this study, there are no benefits to research participation, and the greatest risk to study participation is the loss of confidentiality. To minimize the risk of loss of confidentiality, Ingrid and Estria ask the IRB for a waiver of documentation of consent, in which participants will not sign their name to indicate consent, but rather, consent is implied upon individuals' participation in an interview or focus group (*beneficence*). Also, Ingrid and Estria detail their recruitment procedures and specify that all nurses and prescribers will be eligible to participate (*justice*).

When EBP, Quality Improvement, and Research Converge

In the examples provided, activities neatly exist within an individual category—that is, EBP, quality improvement, or research. Yet, as activities progress and evolve over time in the dynamic clinical arena, their categorization, too, may change and extend beyond a singular category. Real-world examples of the interdependence and overlap among EBP, quality improvement, and research are provided in the following two examples.

CASE STUDY

Scenario

Nurse Michael is a clinical nurse in pediatric outpatient radiology. He finds that magnetic resonance imaging (MRI) can be a stressful event for children. He reviews the published literature for interventions that effectively minimized distress among children undergoing an MRI. He finds that multimodal interventions have successfully reduced distress, but these interventions are resource-intensive and difficult to scale.

Michael engages local leadership to develop a brief educational video on MRI procedures that is tailored for pediatric patients.

Michael wants to formally evaluate the effectiveness of the video on reducing stress. He thinks the video will reduce distress at his institution and thinks children at other institutions might benefit from the video, as well.

Michael discusses his project ideas with the nurse researcher at his institution. After discussing the evolution of the project and the intent of the project, the nurse researcher believes the project meets the definition of research and strongly encourages Michael to submit his intended project to the IRB.

Discussion

Michael was initially interested in implementing interventions that had effectively minimized distress among children undergoing an MRI. After reviewing the literature, Michael found that published interventions could not be feasibly implemented at his institution, and he began developing and evaluating the impact of a new intervention (educational video). Michael wanted to systematically evaluate the impact of the intervention and believed the information gained from his project could be generalizable to other institutions. Thus, while Michael intended to conduct an EBP project, the project evolved into a research study.

Clinical Implications

The categorization of clinical projects may evolve over time. Clinical nurses should be mindful of the criteria that warrant recategorization and make adjustments as necessary.

CASE STUDY

Scenario

Nurse Sarah is a nurse educator in the intensive care unit and leads the interprofessional Pressure Injury Prevention Committee. Sarah and her committee find that the incidence of pressure injuries at their institution is on the rise. They are interested in developing an algorithm to assist nurses at their institution in providing patient-tailored, evidence-based interventions to prevent pressure injuries.

After reviewing the evidence, the group develops an evidence-based algorithm and introduces it at their hospital. To their delight, they find the incidence of pressure injury decreased substantially after the implementation of the algorithm.

The group thinks the algorithm might be effective in preventing pressure injuries at outside institutions and is interested in partnering with outside institutions to evaluate its effectiveness. Sarah and the committee discuss their project ideas with their institution's nurse researcher. After discussing the evolution of the project and the intent of the project, the nurse researcher believes the committee is now interested in conducting research.

Discussion

Sarah and the committee were initially interested in implementing an algorithm to assist nurses at their institution in the implementation of best practices. After observing the impact of the algorithm on the incidence of pressure injuries at their institution, the committee members suspected that the algorithm might be effective in preventing pressure injury at outside institutions and became interested in testing this hypothesis. Thus, while the project began as an EBP project, it morphed into a potential research study.

Clinical Implications

It is important for nurses to thoughtfully consider the nature of their current and anticipated work to ensure that the proper procedures are being followed.

Failure to recognize the morphing of EBP, quality improvement, and research has given way to various myths. One such myth is the belief that only research can be published, which is inaccurate (Office for Human Research Protections, 2016/2020). Such myths perpetuate a belief that EBP, quality improvement, and research exist in mutually exclusive categories, when in fact they are commonly interconnected, as demonstrated in the examples in this chapter. Nurses should continuously appraise their current and anticipated activities to ensure that their projects meet local and federal requirements (if research). The Office for Human

Research Protections of the US Department of Health & Human Services, private universities, and service settings have each developed algorithms and checklists to aid in determining whether activities include research and thus require IRB approval (Children's Hospital of Philadelphia Quality Improvement Committee [QIC] Ethics Subcommittee, 2018; Duke University Health System Human Research Protection Program, 2016; Office for Human Research Protections, 2016/2020). Still, questions may persist, especially as IRB procedures differ between institutions and given the unique nuances of individual projects. Nurses should be encouraged to address areas of uncertainty to their local IRBs and seek guidance from the department of research (or equivalent) at their institutions. Following are some other common myths that clinicians may believe about categorizing clinical research projects.

Common Misconceptions About Clinical Research Categorization

Myth #1
I am doing a quality improvement project for school. Because it's a quality improvement project, I do not need to obtain IRB approval.

Myth #1 Debunked
Not necessarily. There are times when quality improvement projects include research activities, and as such, IRB approval is required.

Myth #2
I am surveying nurses on my unit for a clinical ladder project. Because I am only surveying nurses, I do not need IRB approval.

Myth #2 Debunked
Not necessarily. If the survey is part of research activities, IRB approval is needed.

Myth #3
If I want to publish results from my quality improvement project, I need IRB approval.

Myth #3 Debunked
False. The intent to publish alone does not necessitate IRB approval.

Summary

Nurses are increasingly leading scholarly projects on their clinical units. While scholarly projects may initially be conceived as EBP, quality improvement, or research, such work may evolve to include a combination of activities. To facilitate the conduct of scholarly work that is ethical and methodologically sound, nurses should know of the indications, similarities and differences in EBP, quality improvement, and research and prospectively consider the type of activity they are pursuing to ensure that project procedures are appropriate and meet regulatory requirements. Because the characterization of activities is challenging, nurses should feel encouraged to seek the guidance of local experts.

Review Questions

1. Quality improvement projects do not require IRB approval.
   True or False

   Answer: It depends. Quality improvement activities may include research procedures. It is important for nurses to actively consider their scholarly activities and recognize instances in which IRB approval is needed.

2. Ethical oversight is only needed for research projects. True or False

   Answer: False. All scholarly projects need to be conducted in accordance with ethical principles. The IRB helps ensure that ethical principles are followed in research.

3. The model of EBP at NewYork-Presbyterian Hospital is called _____.

   Answer: PEACE; P = problem identification; E = evidence review; A = appraise evidence; C = conduct research or change practice; E = evaluate and disseminate findings

4. EBP, research, and quality improvement exist along the continuum of clinical scholarship. True or False

   Answer: True. Nurses engage in complementary activities of clinical scholarship with the ultimate goal of improving patient care and outcomes.

5. What are the two criteria of research activities?

   Answer: 1) the activity is designed to contribute to generalizable knowledge, and 2) the activity will be conducted using information gathered from humans.

References

Agency for Healthcare Research and Quality. (2013, May). *Practice facilitation handbook: Module 4. Approaches to quality improvement.* https://www.ahrq.gov/ncepcr/tools/pf-handbook/mod4.html

American Association of Colleges of Nursing. (2008). *The essentials of baccalaureate education for professional nursing practice.* http://www.aacnnursing.org/portals/42/publications/baccessentials08.pdf

Baker, K. M., Clark, P. R., Henderson, D., Wolf, L. A., Carman, M. J., Manton, A., & Zavotsky, K. E. (2014). Identifying the differences between quality improvement, evidence-based practice, and original research. *Journal of Emergency Nursing, 40*(2), 195–197. https://doi.org/10.1016/j.jen.2013.12.016

Boyce, J. M., & Pittet, D. (2002). Guideline for hand hygiene in health-care settings. Recommendations of the Healthcare Infection Control Practices Advisory Committee and the HICPAC/SHEA/APIC/IDSA Hand Hygiene Task Force. *Morbidity and Mortality Weekly Report Recommendations and Reports, 51*(Rr-16), 1–45, quiz CE 41–44. https://www.cdc.gov/mmwr/preview/mmwrhtml/rr5116a1.htm

Carter, E. J., Mastro, K., Vose, C., Rivera, R., & Larson, E. L. (2017). Clarifying the conundrum: Evidence-based practice, quality improvement, or research?: The clinical scholarship continuum. *Journal of Nursing Administration, 47*(5), 266–270. https://journals.lww.com/jonajournal/Abstract/2017/05000/Clarifying_the_Conundrum__Evidence_Based_Practice,.6.aspx

Cato, K. D., Sun, C., Carter, E. J., Liu, J., Rivera, R., & Larson, E. (2019). Linking to improve nursing care and knowledge: Evaluation of an initiative to provide research support to clinical nurses. *Journal of Nursing Administration, 49*(1), 48–54.

Children's Hospital of Philadelphia Quality Improvement Committee (QIC) Ethics Subcommittee. (2018). *CHOP screening checklist for quality improvement (QI) projects.* https://irb.research.chop.edu/sites/default/files/documents/quality_improvement_vs._research_checklist_2018.pdf

Duke University Health System Human Research Protection Program. (2016). *Quality improvement activities in health care versus research.* https://irb.duhs.duke.edu/sites/irb.duhs.duke.edu/files/QI%20policy%20and%20checklist.pdf

Dykes, P. C., Carroll, D. L., Hurley, A., Lipsitz, S., Benoit, A., Chang, F., Meltzer, S., Tsurikova, R., Zuyov, L., & Middleton, B. (2010). Fall prevention in acute care hospitals: A randomized trial. *JAMA, 304*(17), 1912–1918. https://jamanetwork.com/journals/jama/fullarticle/186836

Erasmus, V., Daha, T. J., Brug, H., Richardus, J. H., Behrendt, M. D., Vos, M. C., & van Beeck, E. F. (2010). Systematic review of studies on compliance with hand hygiene guidelines in hospital care. *Infection Control & Hospital Epidemiology, 31*(3), 283–294.

Fitzpatrick, J. J. (2016). Distinctions between research, evidence based practice, and quality improvement. *Applied Nursing Research, 29*, 261.

Grady, C. (2018). Ethical principles in clinical research. In J. I. Gallin, F. P. Ognibene, & L. L. Johnson (Eds.), *Principles and practice of clinical research* (4th ed., pp. 19–31). Academic Press.

Institute of Medicine (US) Committee on the Health Professions Education Summit, Greiner, A. C., & Knebel, E. (2003). The core competencies needed for health care professionals. In *Health professions education: A bridge to quality*. National Academies Press. https://www.ncbi.nlm.nih.gov/books/NBK221519/

Lambe, K. A., Lydon, S., Madden, C., Vellinga, A., Hehir, A., Walsh, M., & O'Connor, P. (2019). Hand hygiene compliance in the ICU: A systematic review. *Critical Care Medicine, 47*(9), 1251–1257. https://doi.org/10.1097/CCM.0000000000003868

Office for Human Research Protections. (2016/2020). *Human subject regulations decision charts*. https://www.hhs.gov/ohrp/regulations-and-policy/decision-charts/index.html

Pittet, D., Allegranzi, B., & Boyce, J. (2009). The World Health Organization guidelines on hand hygiene in health care and their consensus recommendations. *Infection Control & Hospital Epidemiology, 30*(7), 611–622. https://doi.org/10.1086/600379

Powell, K. (2015). Nursing research: Nurses know best. *Nature, 522*(7557), 507–509. https://doi.org/10.1038/nj7557-507a

Sackett, D. L., Rosenberg, W. M., Gray, J. A., Haynes, R. B., & Richardson, W. S. (1996). Evidence based medicine: What it is and what it isn't. *BMJ, 312*(7023), 71–72. https://doi.org/10.1136/bmj.312.7023.71

Shirey, M. R., Hauck, S. L., Embree, J. L., Kinner, T. J., Schaar, G. L., Phillips, L. A., Ashby, S. R., Swenty, C. F., & McCool, I. A. (2011). Showcasing differences between quality improvement, evidence-based practice, and research. *Journal of Continuing Education in Nursing, 42*(2), 57–68; quiz 69–70.

Slutsman, J., & Nieman, L. (2018). Institutional review boards. In J. I. Gallin, F. P. Ognibene, & L. L. Johnson (Eds.), *Principles and practice of clinical research* (4th ed., pp. 47–61). Academic Press.

Stevens, K. R. (2013). The impact of evidence-based practice in nursing and the next big ideas. *Online Journal of Issues in Nursing, 18*(2), 4.

Tahan, H. M., Rivera, R. R., Carter, E. J., Gallagher, K. A., Fitzpatrick, J. J., & Manzano, W. M. (2016). Evidence-based nursing practice: The PEACE framework. *Nurse Leader, 14*(1), 57–61. https://doi.org/10.1016/j.mnl.2015.07.012

PEACE MODEL

P | **PROBLEM IDENTIFICATION**
Formulate the clinical question (**PICO**):
- **P** | Patient Population
- **I** | Intervention
- **C** | Comparison of Intervention
- **O** | Outcome

E | **EVIDENCE REVIEW**
Review evidence relevant to your clinical question by searching databases.

A | **APPRAISE EVIDENCE**
Appraise the evidence that appears highest in the hierarchy of scientific evidence for its quality and applicability to practice.

C | **CHANGE PRACTICE OR CONDUCT RESEARCH**
If evidence is sufficient, embark on improvement project to address practice change.

If evidence is insufficient to warrant practice change, conduct research.

E | **EVALUATE AND DISSEMINATE FINDINGS**
Evaluate the impact of the implemented practice change and research results.

Disseminate findings through publication, oral, and poster presentations.

2

PROBLEM IDENTIFICATION

–Bevin Cohen, PhD, MS, MPH, RN

KEYWORDS | PHRASES

PICO question, evidence-based practice, literature search

CHAPTER OBJECTIVES

After studying this chapter, learners will be able to:

1. Describe the P of the PEACE model.
2. Explain the components of PICO questions: Problem, intervention, comparison, and outcome.
3. Given a clinical scenario, identify the PICO question.

Introduction

One morning during rounds on an inpatient gynecological oncology unit, an experienced nurse paused to think. The patient in front of her had a drainage percutaneous endoscopic gastrostomy tube (dPEG) placed the previous morning, and she would have new dietary orders for the next few days. This scenario was not new or unusual to the nurse. In fact, many patients on this unit with advanced ovarian cancer opt for dPEGs to alleviate symptoms of malignant bowel obstruction (Rath et al., 2013; Zucchi et al., 2016). Still, looking around the room at her colleagues, the nurse came to a disquieting realization. Many clinicians ordered liquid diets for patients with dPEGs due to the terrible nausea, vomiting, and cramping patients can experience after eating solid foods—even soft ones. However, a few clinicians on the unit ordered a range of diets for patients with dPEGs. The nurse silently wondered if perhaps this was the reason why she was frequently managing patients with dPEGs who were unable to tolerate their diets. In her notepad she jotted down a question to investigate after the morning chaos quieted. It read, "What is the recommended diet for patients after dPEG placement?"

As a diligent clinician, the nurse checked the hospital policy on dPEG management later that day. Scanning through the document, she came upon the section for diet and nutrition. She read the section carefully and was surprised to find that her question was only partially answered. The policy stated that patients should remain on clear liquids for 48 hours following dPEG placement, but after that there was no definitive guidance—patients could move to full liquids, pureed foods, or solid foods at the discretion of the clinician. Wanting to improve patients' gastrointestinal symptoms and alleviate their suffering, the nurse went in search of evidence that could help guide dietary orders for patients with dPEGs.

The nurse began by returning to the question she had written down in her notebook. "What is the recommended diet for patients after dPEG placement?" During her lunch break she visited the hospital's medical library and typed the phrase into an internet search engine. A flood of results returned, but none were particularly helpful. There were many patient-facing educational materials and instructions for dPEG care at home, and although they contained ample guidance on eating and drinking, the guidance varied from institution to institution and lacked references to scientific literature. In search of scientific peer-reviewed literature, the nurse opened a new tab and searched the same phrase in PubMed. This time she was inundated with thousands of articles about all types of percutaneous endoscopic gastrostomy tubes for all sorts of indications, seemingly in no particular order and with no particular relation to dietary management for oncology patients with palliative dPEGs to manage malignant bowel obstruction. Frustrated, the nurse then remembered something she had learned during her bachelor's degree program: a systematic method for honing a clinical question by breaking it down into its key components—the PICO framework.

The PICO Question

The PICO question is designed to help clinicians effectively search the literature to answer clinical questions and serves as the basis for evidence-based practice (EBP). EBP movements are based on the premise that patient outcomes could be improved if clinicians routinely consulted, critically appraised, and incorporated relevant knowledge gathered from the best available evidence to supplement their clinical judgment, which is developed over time through didactic training, firsthand experience, and clinical observations (Guyatt et al., 1992; Smith & Rennie, 2014). To effectively implement EBP, clinicians need a systematic and reliable method for identifying the relevant evidence. This process begins with asking the right clinical question (Schardt et al., 2007). The PICO framework helps clinicians create focused clinical questions by breaking the questions down into four key components (Richardson et al., 1995):

P **Population**—What is the patient population of interest?

I **Intervention**—What is the intervention in question?

C **Comparison**—What is the alternative approach to which the intervention is being compared?

O **Outcome**—What is the outcome that the intervention is intended to address?

Let us return to the nurse and her question, "What is the recommended diet for patients after dPEG placement?" This type of question is an appropriate starting place for clinicians who are searching for practice guidelines or institutional policies. However, this example illustrates a common situation in which no cohesive or current guideline can be found. In cases like this, clinicians must turn to the literature to identify, critically appraise, and synthesize relevant findings themselves to guide their practice.

Because the nurse in this example was unable to identify a clinical practice guideline to answer her question, she had to change her approach. After searching "What is the recommended diet for patients after dPEG placement?" in PubMed, which returned an unfocused deluge of articles, the nurse employed the PICO framework to hone her clinical question and perform a more effective search. She began by identifying the population, intervention, comparison, and outcome as follows:

P **Population**—Patients with cancer

I **Intervention**—Liquid diet

C **Comparison**—Pureed

O **Outcome**—Nausea and vomiting

PICO question: For patients with cancer, is a liquid diet more effective than a pureed diet for preventing nausea and vomiting?

The nurse conducted a literature search using keywords for each of the four elements and retrieved a large number of articles. The titles and abstracts seemed no closer to answering her question, and she quickly realized why: Nowhere in her

PICO question did she specify that she was interested in dietary intervention for patients with dPEGs. Realizing that her population was more specific than "patients with cancer," she revised her PICO question as follows:

P   **Population**—Patients with drainage percutaneous endoscopic gastrostomy

I   **Intervention**—Liquid diet

C   **Comparison**—Pureed diet

O   **Outcome**—Nausea and vomiting

PICO question: For patients with drainage percutaneous endoscopic gastrostomy, is a liquid diet more effective than a pureed diet for preventing nausea and vomiting?

Narrowing the focus of the population helped to narrow the search results, but the vast majority of studies seemed to focus on nutritional management for patients with percutaneous endoscopic gastrostomy for indications other than drainage, the indication for placement in patients with malignant bowel obstruction. Again, she refined her PICO question:

P   **Population**—Patients with drainage percutaneous endoscopic gastrostomy for management of malignant bowel obstruction

I   **Intervention**—Liquid diet

C   **Comparison**—Pureed diet

O   **Outcome**—Nausea and vomiting

PICO question: For patients with drainage percutaneous endoscopic gastrostomy for management of malignant bowel obstruction, is a liquid diet more effective than a pureed diet for preventing nausea and vomiting?

Steps in Forming the PICO Question

Developing a PICO question is often an iterative process, whereby the clinician refines each element of a clinical question—population (in whom?), intervention (through what means?), comparison (compared to what?), and outcome (to what end?)—to focus the question and narrow search results to the evidence that is best suited to answer it in a particular practice setting.

Population: In Whom?

The first step when reviewing the literature is to carefully define the **population (P)** of interest. Suppose, for example, that a nurse working in a pediatric outpatient specialty clinic wants to know whether self-management interventions are beneficial for improving asthma control. Because the nurse works in a pediatric practice, he conducts a literature search focusing on the population of "pediatrics." He gets many results, but the findings are mixed, and the interventions seem to be tailored toward specific age groups and developmental stages within the pediatric population. Knowing that his clinic is focused on improving asthma control for school-age children, the nurse narrows his population of interest to children 6 to 12 years old and conducts the search again. This time the results and interventions are much more consistent, though there is still some heterogeneity in the patient populations under study: Some interventions focus on supporting self-management for children with newly diagnosed asthma, whereas others focus on long-term self-management for children who have lived with asthma for years. Some focus on children who have already taken an active role in managing their disease, whereas others focus on children who are transitioning into assuming more management responsibilities once held by their parent or caregiver. Further still, the nurse was able to divide the articles into those that focused on children who were novice with using medication versus those that focused on children who were experts (Lozano & Houtrow, 2018). Narrowing the population from *pediatric patients* to *school-age patients who are newly diagnosed with asthma and novice at disease and medication management* helps ensure that the nurse's literature search will retrieve studies that were conducted in the same population in which the nurse intends to implement a self-management intervention. This is a critical step in the PICO process because many interventions work differently in different populations. In this example, it is easy to imagine that a self-management mobile health app that is effective in young adults might not be effective for school-age children due to differences in reading comprehension, access to technology, and cognitive ability to understand medication management algorithms. Similarly, the information and learning needs of a child newly diagnosed with asthma may far exceed those of a child who is the same age but has lived with asthma for her whole life.

Intervention: Through What Means?

Most clinical inquiries naturally begin with a question about whether a particular **intervention (I)** is the best method for achieving a particular outcome in a given population or setting. In nursing, medicine, and the allied health professions, interventions tend to be modified, refined, and adapted to new uses, settings, and patient populations over time. Therefore, formulating a PICO question that includes a narrowly specified intervention is helpful for arriving at the appropriate clinical question and performing an effective literature search. In this scenario, the nurse begins with the intervention *asthma medication self-management*, and thousands of articles examining the effects of a wide range of self-management interventions are returned. The nurse reviews the results and notices, for example, self-management interventions stemming from medical provider-driven models, collaborative models, and self-agency models (Rangachari, 2017). Some articles test self-management approaches centered on written personalized action plans, whereas others test approaches centered on facilitating greater access to consultation with healthcare professionals between scheduled office visits (Pinnock, 2015). Knowing that his practice does not currently use personalized written asthma action plans, the nurse chooses to focus his PICO question on the efficacy of this intervention and changes the phrase *asthma medication self-management* to the more specific *personalized written asthma action plan*.

Comparison: Compared to What?

When considering whether an intervention will have a beneficial effect in a particular setting, the nurse must consider the alternative approaches to which it is being compared. In most studies, interventions are compared to either usual care—that is, the standard practices that are already in place at the institution at the time of the study—or an alternative intervention. In this scenario, the nurse is interested in whether implementing a new intervention—personalized written asthma action plans—will improve asthma control among patients in his clinic. Therefore, he focuses his PICO question to include a **comparison (C)** that reflects the current standard of care in his clinic, which is *personalized education*.

Outcome: To What End?

The final element of a focused PICO question is a narrowly defined **outcome (O)**. In this scenario, the nurse begins his inquiry with the overarching goal of improving asthma control in children. After reviewing the results of a handful of studies, the nurse realizes that *asthma control* is a construct that can have many definitions and is composed of many components. To effectively compare results across studies, it is important to focus on outcome measures that have clear definitions and methods of measurement. Asthma control can be measured in terms of functional status such as pulmonary function or ability to participate in routine exercise; healthcare utilization such as emergency department (ED) visits or hospitalizations; or other measures such as quality of life or asthma-related mortality. An intervention may have an effect on one or many of these outcomes. However, asking whether an intervention improves quality of life formulates a different PICO question than, for example, asking whether an intervention reduces ED visits. Focusing the PICO question on a single outcome or a group of closely related outcomes helps ensure that the clinician will be able to effectively summarize the available evidence. In this example, the nurse chooses to focus on the outcome of *unplanned clinic visits*, which are common in his practice. He performs a literature search using the PICO question, "For school-age patients who are newly diagnosed with asthma and novice at disease and medication management, are personalized written asthma action plans more effective than personalized education for reducing clinic visits?"

Why Ask Why?

Speaking up about practice concerns can be difficult for all healthcare workers and for nurses in particular (Okuyama et al., 2014). In some practice settings, challenging the status quo and questioning "the way we've always done it here" can be viewed by peers and supervisors as naïve, trouble-making, or insubordinate (Bloom, 2018; Townsend, 2016; Zolnierek, 2012). As a result, nurses may be unwilling to raise new ideas or concerns about current practices for fear of retaliation or because they feel that administrators will not consider their comments (Cole et al., 2019; Dinndorf-Hogenson, 2015; Okuyama et al., 2014).

So is it worth it to "rock the boat?" The evidence shows that it is and that doing so contributes to a healthy team dynamic, patient safety culture, and improved outcomes for patients (Kolbe et al., 2012; Lefton, 2013; Okuyama et al., 2014). As patient advocates, nurses should feel empowered to ask questions about whether current practices in their institution align with the best available evidence (American Nurses Association, 2015; Zolnierek, 2012). A critical part of being an effective advocate is being able to articulate clinical problems and propose possible alternatives that are evidence-based (Zolnierek, 2012).

Even when institutions have developed robust policies, protocols, or practice guidelines based on the best available evidence and expert review, it is important to recognize that science is not static, and new information is constantly emerging. In the United States alone there were more than 4 million original articles published and indexed in PubMed from 1999 through 2015, with the annual total nearly tripling from approximately 130,000 to approximately 330,000 articles during that 20-year time frame (Fontelo & Liu, 2018). Therefore, it is important for nurses and administrators to frequently revisit current practices and review any new literature that may provide updated guidance. Furthermore, even with evidence-based guidelines in place, it is important to keep in mind that the effects of interventions may differ across populations. As established practices are tested in new environments, differences in efficacy across populations may come to light. Choosing the appropriate "P" (population) during the PICO process helps to guide a review of the evidence that is tailored to a specific patient population or practice area, which may reveal different evidence-based strategies than those included in a general policy or guideline.

Summary

New knowledge about best practices is constantly evolving. Patients are best served when nurses and other allied health professionals continuously reassess practice standards to ensure they are aligned with the best available evidence. The PICO framework aids clinicians with formulating clear and specific questions that guide evidence review. A well-formulated PICO question allows clinicians to compare outcomes associated with different interventions for a given population and choose the most appropriate practice to implement in their setting.

Review Questions

Scenario for Questions 1–3

A nurse just transferred to a different medical-surgical unit in his hospital. The medical-surgical unit where he used to work followed an hourly rounding protocol to prevent patient falls, and he felt it was effective for this purpose. He is surprised that his new unit does not follow the same policy and wants to suggest it to his manager. However, he realized that, although he felt the policy prevented falls based on his experience, he had no clinical evidence to support his hunch. The nurse decides to review the literature prior to discussing the policy with his manager. He begins his search by asking, "Is hourly rounding effective for patients on medical-surgical units?"

1. What are the elements of PICO that are missing from the nurse's question?
    Answer: comparison and outcome

2. Rewrite the PICO question to incorporate the missing elements.
    Answer: For patients on medical-surgical units, is hourly rounding more effective than relying on call bells for preventing falls?

3. If the nurse's search delivers a large number of results, what could he do to improve the relevance of the articles to his unit?

    Answer: He could define the P (population) more narrowly. For example, if his unit had many patients with delirium, he could change the population to *patients with delirium on medical-surgical units.*

Scenario for Questions 4 and 5

A patient asks her postpartum nurse about whether she should co-sleep with her newborn infant or have the infant sleep in a separate bassinette. The nurse knows that co-sleeping is a controversial topic and that recommendations about co-sleeping continue to evolve. She wants to give her patient the best available evidence to make an informed decision. She and her patient both read recently that co-sleeping may be helpful for successful breastfeeding, but on the other hand, it may increase the risk of sudden infant death syndrome (SIDS).

4. How might the nurse search the literature for possible pros and cons of co-sleeping using PICO?

    Answer: Because the patient and nurse have questions about possible pros and cons of co-sleeping—successful breastfeeding and SIDS—the nurse could formulate two separate PICO questions, each with a different O (outcome).

5. Write the PICO strategy that the nurse could use to search the literature.

    Answer: Do newborn infants who co-sleep have a higher risk of SIDS compared with newborn infants who sleep in a separate bassinette? And, are newborn infants who co-sleep more likely to be successful breast feeders compared with newborn infants who sleep in a separate bassinette?

References

American Nurses Association. (2015). *Nursing: Scope and standards of practice* (3rd ed.). American Nurses Association.

Bloom, E. M. (2018). Horizontal violence among nurses: Experiences, responses, and job performance. *Nursing Forum, 51,* 77–83. https://doi.org/10.1111/nuf.12300

Cole, D. A., Bersick, E., Skarbek, A., Cummins, K., Dugan, K., & Grantoza, R. (2019). The courage to speak out: A study describing nurses' attitudes to report unsafe practices in patient care. *Journal of Nursing Management, 27*(6), 1176–1181. https://doi.org/10.1111/jonm.12789

Dinndorf-Hogenson, G. A. (2015). Moral courage in practice: Implications for patient safety. *Journal of Nursing Regulation, 6*(2), 10–16. https://doi.org/10.1016/S2155-8256(15)30381-1

Fontelo, P., & Liu, F. (2018). A review of recent publication trends from top publishing countries. *Systematic Reviews, 7*, 147. https://doi.org/10.1186/s13643-018-0819-1

Guyatt, G., Cairns, J., Churchill, D., Cook, D., Haynes, B., Hirsh, J., Irvine, J., Levine, M., Levine, M., Nishikawa, J., Sackett, D., Brill-Edwards, P., Gerstein, H., Gibson, J., Jaeschke, R., Kerigan, A., Neville, A., Panju, A., Detsky, A., . . . Tugwell, P. (1992). Evidence-based medicine: A new approach to teaching the practice of medicine. *Journal of the American Medical Association, 268*(17), 2420–2425. https://doi.org/10.1001/jama.1992.03490170092032

Kolbe, M., Burtscher, M. J., Wacker, J., Grande, B., Nohynkova, R., Manser, T., Spahn, D. R., & Grote, G. (2012). Speaking up is related to better performance in simulated anesthesia inductions: An observational study. *Anesthesia and Analgesia, 115*, 1099–1108. https://doi.org/10.1213/ANE.0b013e318269cd32

Lefton, C. (2013). Why disruption can be a good thing. *American Nurse Today, 8*(5). https://www.americannursetoday.com/why-disruption-can-be-a-good-thing/

Lozano, P., & Houtrow, A. (2018). Supporting self-management in children and adolescents with complex chronic conditions. *Pediatrics, 141*, S233–S241. https://doi.org/10.1542/peds.2017-1284H

Okuyama, A., Wagner, C., & Bijnen, B. (2014). Speaking up for patient safety by hospital-based health care professionals: A literature review. *BMC Health Services Research, 14*, 61. https://doi.org/10.1186/1472-6963-14-61

Pinnock, H. (2015). Supported self-management for asthma. *Breathe, 11*(2), 98–109. https://doi.org/10.1183/20734735.015614

Rangachari, P. (2017). A framework for measuring self-management effectiveness and health care use among pediatric asthma patients and families. *Journal of Asthma and Allergy, 10*, 111–112. https://doi.org/10.2147/JAA.S133481

Rath, K. S., Loseth, D., Muscarella, P., Phillips, G. S., Fowler, J. M., O'Malley, D. M., Cohn, D. E., Copeland, L. J., Eisenhauer, E. L., & Salani, R. (2013). Outcomes following percutaneous upper gastrointestinal decompressive tube placement for malignant bowel obstruction in ovarian cancer. *Gynecological Oncology, 129*, 103–106. https://doi.org/10.1016/j.ygyno.2013.01.021

Richardson, W. S., Wilson, M. C., Nishikawa, J., & Hayward, R. S. A. (1995). The well-built clinical question: A key to evidence-based decisions. *American College of Physicians Journal Club, 123*, A12. https://doi.org/10.7326/ACPJC-1995-123-3-A12

Schardt, C., Adams, M. B., Owens, T., Keitz, S., & Fontelo, P. (2007). Utilization of the PICO framework to improve searching PubMed for clinical questions. *BMC Medical Informatics and Decision Making, 7*, 16. https://doi.org/10.1186/1472-6947-7-16

Smith, R., & Rennie, D. (2014). Evidence based medicine—an oral history. The British *Medical Journal, 348*, g371. https://doi.org/10.1136/bmj.g371

Townsend, T. (2016). Not just "eating our young": Workplace bullying strikes experienced nurses, too. *American Nurse Today, 11*(2). https://www.americannursetoday.com/just-eating-young-workplace-bullying-strikes-experienced-nurses/

Zolnierek, C. (2012). Speak to be heard: Effective nurse advocacy. *American Nurse Today, 7*(10). https://www.americannursetoday.com/speak-to-be-heard-effective-nurse-advocacy/

Zucchi, E., Fornasarig, M., Martella, L., Maiero, S., Lucia, E., Borsatti, E., Balestreri, L., Giorda, G., Annunziata, M. A., & Cannizzaro, R. (2016). Decompressive percutaneous endoscopic gastrostomy in advanced cancer patients with small-bowel obstruction is feasible and effective: A large prospective study. *Supportive Care in Cancer, 24*, 2877–2882. https://doi.org/10.1007/s00520-016-3102-9

PEACE MODEL

P

PROBLEM IDENTIFICATION

Formulate the clinical question (**PICO**):

- **P** | Patient Population
- **I** | Intervention
- **C** | Comparison of Intervention
- **O** | Outcome

E

EVIDENCE REVIEW

Review evidence relevant to your clinical question by searching databases.

A

APPRAISE EVIDENCE

Appraise the evidence that appears highest in the hierarchy of scientific evidence for its quality and applicability to practice.

C

CHANGE PRACTICE OR CONDUCT RESEARCH

If evidence is sufficient, embark on improvement project to address practice change.

If evidence is insufficient to warrant practice change, conduct research.

E

EVALUATE AND DISSEMINATE FINDINGS

Evaluate the impact of the implemented practice change and research results.

Disseminate findings through publication, oral, and poster presentations.

EVIDENCE REVIEW

-Keith C. Mages, PhD, MLS, MSN, RN, AHIP

KEYWORDS | PHRASES
literature search, databases, evidence-based practice, quality improvement, research, MeSH, PubMed, Medline, tables of evidence, citation management

CHAPTER OBJECTIVES

After studying this chapter, learners will be able to:

1. Describe the E of the PEACE model.
2. Identify the specific search needs required for EBP projects, QI activities, and research studies.
3. Identify important nursing and biomedical databases and develop effective literature search strategies.

Introduction

Once a clinical or research question is identified, the next step in the PEACE model is evidence review (Tahan et al., 2016). Nurses interested in increasing their health knowledge can turn to a diverse assortment of online resources when investigating topics of interest. While the results of a simple Google search may suffice at times, nurses intending to contribute to the research process will need to develop their searching skills in additional, more specialized resources such as PubMed, CINAHL, and Cochrane. This chapter delivers a comprehensive overview of the literature search process, including:

- Search needs specific to evidence-based practice, quality improvement, and research projects
- Literature search development and PICO questions

- Common biomedical and nursing-specific databases
- Nuts and bolts of literature searching
- Management of evidence retrieved

Relevant Evidence: Identifying Search Needs Specific to EBP Projects, QI Activities, and Research Studies

As discussed in Chapter 1, nurses typically conduct investigative initiatives classified in one of three ways: evidence-based practice projects, quality improvement activities, and research studies. Each of these project/initiative/study types has different aims and goals, and likewise, each requires different considerations during the evidence review process.

Evidence-Based Practice Evidence Review

Evidence-based practice (EBP) translates the best available evidence on a particular topic into impactful clinical decision-making (Conner, 2014). Therefore, the first step in any successful EBP project is the acquisition of quality, clinically relevant evidence. Literature used for EBP projects tends to be based on recent publications, produced in the past 5 to 10 years (Spurlock, 2019). While a seminal, older article on a particular topic may indeed be referenced, results are typically limited to newer data to ensure the evidence analyzed is truly representative of current clinical knowledge. EBP projects tend to rely on evidence summaries and guidelines more than other types of investigations. These specific types of references provide comprehensive overviews of available high-quality evidence on a particular topic, optimally compiling information from multiple systematic reviews to recommend only the most impactful interventions available (Agoritsas et al., 2015).

Common EBP resources that provide evidence summaries include UpToDate (www.uptodate.com) and DynaMed (https://www.dynamed.com/home/). Both resources synthesize a multitude of clinical topics; however, each structures summaries differently. UpToDate tends to structure summaries in a chapter-like fashion, whereas DynaMed favors presenting its information in bullet point format. Initially developed to address the needs of the nursing profession, the Joanna Briggs

Institute EBP Database (Ovid; https://joannabriggs.org/ebp#database) provides another option for EBP evidence summaries. It is important to note, however, that each of these databases requires individual or institutional subscriptions to access the evidence summaries. If interested, it is recommended that you check with your institutional library prior to purchasing a subscription, as unfortunately each of these can be quite costly.

Clinical guidelines offer another route to explore while preparing for EBP endeavors. Unlike evidence summaries, these sources of information tend to be freely available, produced by professional health organizations or government bodies. Clinical guidelines provide overviews of clinical topics of specific importance to the authoring bodies and are typically published in affiliated journals or on organizational and governmental webpages (Agoritsas et al., 2015). At one time, the U.S. National Guideline Clearinghouse (https://www.ahrq.gov/gam/index.html) provided a convenient, comprehensive means to search clinical guidelines; however, as of 2018 this important resource lost funding from the national government and is consequently no longer updated. It is mentioned here as background information, as this database is still commonly referenced in the literature and by researchers. To locate clinical guidelines today, simply Googling a topic of interest followed by "clinical guideline" may also be a worthwhile search, as many clinical guidelines are published openly on freely accessible webpages. One might also consider visiting the organizational webpages of interest to search for any available topical guidelines. Of course, a more systematic way of searching for guidelines exists via PubMed, the National Library of Medicine's popular and freely available MEDLINE platform (https://www.ncbi.nlm.nih.gov/pubmed/). See the PubMed section later in this chapter for further information on how to locate clinical guidelines in this manner.

When searching, you may discover a lack of gold-standard clinical summaries or guidelines. This could be because there is a lack of high-quality data available to create these summaries or because a more obscure (or newer) topic has not yet been addressed adequately by the research community. In these cases, individual systematic reviews or randomized controlled trials may be necessary to consult. However, these specific results may not be easily translated into practice. If the best evidence discovered is not of sufficient quality or is based on a population or setting different from the one of interest, it may be necessary to pause the implementation of new EBP projects until more sufficient evidence is discovered (Bernhofer, 2015). In this case, enterprising nurses may choose to implement a traditional research study instead to elevate the quality of available literature.

Quality Improvement Evidence Review

Quality Improvement (QI) activities focus on addressing a local need within a particular healthcare setting. QI activities aim to improve specific administrative processes or patient outcomes on a unit level and as such are typically not intended to produce generalizable knowledge (Conner, 2014). Due to their more limited scope, the literature review portion of such projects may be less intensive than those necessary for EBP or research endeavors. However, an adequate review and appraisal of available evidence is still a vital component of the QI process.

Fundamental to these activities is the belief that an alternative process may be superior to current practice. Literature investigating both existing practice and any proposed changes should therefore be explored. Simply because an intervention is initiated in one setting does not mean that it can be safely or successfully implemented elsewhere. Current, peer-reviewed literature should be located to support the practice being proposed. Common databases consulted during QI evidence review include PubMed, CINAHL, and Cochrane. Other databases may also be consulted, particularly if the QI project looks at phenomena typically outside of the biomedical realm. For instance, ERIC may be consulted for educational literature, just as PsycINFO may be analyzed for information specific to mental health or behavioral health knowledge.

A caveat when researching QI activities: If the evidence gathered identifies potential risks of a proposed practice, it may be necessary to shift gears on the activity. In this instance, you may want to consult your Institutional Review Board, as the project may necessarily progress to a more labor-intensive research study (Bernhofer, 2015).

Evidence Review for Research Studies

At their core, research studies seek to produce new knowledge. Researchers may also seek to validate existing knowledge. Paramount in such endeavors is the use of the scientific method to systematically test generated hypotheses (Conner, 2014). A thorough evaluation of available, relevant background literature sets the stage for future discoveries and as such is an important component of any scientifically minded research study. Typically, literature searches performed in support of research studies are broader than those for EBP projects or QI activities (Spurlock, 2019). Information may be gained from systematic reviews and randomized controlled trials, but the researcher may also learn from case reports, editorials, letters to the editor, dissertations, and conference proceedings. A diverse assortment of sources provides valuable perspective and helps inform the researcher on the current state of knowledge regarding the phenomenon of interest: *What is known thus far? What methods have been used to study the topic? What controversies, challenges, and gaps have been reported by other researchers?* Only after these questions are addressed through synthesis of current, pertinent literature can researchers identify the ideal path forward for their research study (Bernhofer, 2015).

Literature Search Development and PICO Questions

Although the type of project undertaken may necessitate different types of literature, a well-crafted question serves as the entry point to successful literature searches, regardless of project type (Carman et al., 2013). PICO questions, composed of **P**opulation/**P**atient, **I**ntervention/**E**xposure, **C**omparison, and **O**utcome elements, can help identify initial search terms (Robb & Shellenbarger, 2014).

For example, consider the following PICO question:

> *Among adult patients with a diagnosis of congestive heart failure (P), how do low health literacy levels (I; in this case more of an E or exposure [to low levels of literacy]) compared to adequate health literacy levels (C) impact patient mortality (O)?*

From this example, we can easily pinpoint several concepts important to our research question, including: *adult, patients, congestive heart failure, health literacy,* and *mortality.* These keywords form the essential components of a literature search and break our question into smaller components that are more compatible with traditional database searching methods (Ho et al., 2016). It may help to take a few minutes to consider each of the key concepts in your PICO questions and develop a list of synonyms, acronyms, or spelling variations for each (Gerberi & Shirk Marienau, 2017). For example, *congestive heart failure* may also be referred to as *CHF, cardiac failure, left-sided heart failure, right-sided heart failure, heart decompensation,* and *myocardial failure.*

Developing a search from your PICO question doesn't only make the literature review process easier, it also helps ensure better results. Research has shown that using PICO as a search strategy development tool increases the sensitivity (the identification of pertinent results) of literature searches (Eriksen & Frandsen, 2018). In general, the more terms identified, the greater the amount of potentially relevant results retrieved.

Common Biomedical and Nursing Databases

With the basic concepts of your literature search identified, it is time to begin searching pertinent databases. Toward this end, a basic knowledge of the types of databases available, as well as the similarities and differences of each, can help to make your searching experience less time-consuming and more fruitful. Consider also consulting with a librarian, nurse researcher, or nurse educator during these early stages. Their insights regarding recommended search terms and databases can help streamline the searching process considerably.

Commonly used databases in the nursing, biomedical, and social science fields are presented in Table 3.1.

Primary Literature Databases

To ensure adequate retrieval of evidence, multiple databases should be consulted. Databases such as Medline, CINAHL, PsycINFO, ERIC, and EMBASE index thousands of professional journals specific to particular subject domains. These databases provide a systematic way to search and identify individual journal article citations, providing access to abstracts (when available) and links to full text (again, when available). In this way, they are excellent resources to access primary literature sources (also referred to as *unfiltered literature*). Randomized controlled trials, epidemiologic studies, qualitative studies, and case reports are among the kinds of literature typically indexed in these databases. This delineation is not absolute, however, as many of these resources do provide access to secondary literature such as systematic reviews and meta-analyses. However, the bulk of citations included in these types of databases tend to be the outcome of more traditional research endeavors, aimed at developing new scientific knowledge.

Medline

Established by the U.S. National Library of Medicine (NLM), Medline is a biomedical database that contains over 25 million biomedical references (U.S. National Library of Medicine, n.d.). Like many databases, Medline can be accessed in multiple ways, via different platforms.

PubMed

PubMed is one such platform, or access point. Like Medline, PubMed is also developed by the NLM. You may see the terms PubMed and Medline used interchangeably, although this is not correct. PubMed is the free platform through which researchers can access the Medline database. Unique to PubMed is Clinical Queries, a tool that automatically applies highly specific filters to search results and rapidly connects researchers to clinically relevant etiologic, diagnostic, therapeutic, or prognostic papers or to systematic reviews (PubMed Clinical Queries, n.d.).

Ovid

Ovid, a Wolters Kluwer platform, also provides access to Medline (Ovid Medline, n.d.). When accessing Medline via Ovid, researchers typically use the term Ovid Medline. Because PubMed is freely available, researchers may wonder why one might use Ovid Medline, which requires a subscription to use. The main difference between these two platforms is the search mechanics. Some users prefer the more detailed searching enabled by the Ovid platform, as compared to the more automated searching techniques used by PubMed. More specifics about these differences are covered later in this chapter. It should be noted that the Ovid platform also provides access to other databases, such as EMBASE, PsycINFO, and ERIC. If your institution has a subscription to Ovid, this platform offers a convenient means of searching multiple databases efficiently.

CINAHL

CINAHL, the Cumulative Index to Nursing and Allied Health Literature, provides citations for over 6 million nursing and allied health publications from nursing journals, the National League for Nursing, and the American Nurses Association (CINAHL Database, n.d.). It is considered the premier database for nursing knowledge and should be an essential resource to consult prior to any nursing research study.

PsycINFO

PsycINFO is a database of the American Psychological Association (APA), which indexes journals, dissertations, and books specific to the behavioral and social sciences (PsycINFO, n.d.). This highly specialized database is essential when researching topics in the field of mental health and includes historical literature as far back as the 1880s.

Web of Science

Web of Science is a very large, multidisciplinary collection of databases with over 1.6 billion references (Web of Science, n.d.). An especially useful feature of Web of Science is citation tracking, including the ability to organize results according to the number of times a paper has been cited. This makes it an excellent resource when looking to gauge a particular article's scholarly impact. Similarly, Web of Science also provides access to Journal Citation Reports, which determines journal impact factor, and provides journal impact rankings based on subject area (Web of Science Group, n.d.).

ERIC

ERIC, or Education Resources Information Center, is a freely available database developed by the Institute of Education Sciences of the U.S. Department of Education. ERIC indexes education research found in journal articles, books, and *grey literature* (citations from sources outside of journals or other traditional scholarship; ERIC content, n.d.). This coverage includes nursing and health science educational literature. When investigating patient or health professional learning styles, ERIC is a database that may warrant consideration.

EMBASE

EMBASE is another biomedical database, similar to Medline in scope of content. EMBASE features over 32 million records and indexes over 8,000 journals, including approximately 2,900 journals not included in Medline (Embase content, n.d.). EMBASE also indexes many conference proceedings and abstracts and as such is a good place to go when looking for grey literature.

Secondary Literature Databases

Databases such as the Cochrane Library, JBI Evidence-Based Database, UpTo-Date, and DynaMed provide coverage of secondary or filtered literature—that is, references developed from multiple primary resources. Primarily these types of databases provide access to syntheses of scientific data and index and provide access to systematic reviews/meta-analyses or EBP topic summaries. As such, they often contain data that can inform clinical decisions and be more easily integrated into current practice. It is important to note that the production of filtered literature tends to be labor intensive and necessarily derived from multiple scientifically sound primary research studies. As such, these particular databases typically contain far fewer records than their unfiltered counterparts. There is not always enough time or quality research available to support the production of filtered literature. Therefore, searchers who do not locate their topic of interest in these databases should also search one or more of the primary literature databases described in the previous section to ensure an adequate review of the literature.

The Cochrane Library

The Cochrane Library provides access to several databases, the most well known of which is the Cochrane Database of Systematic Reviews. The systematic reviews featured in the Cochrane Library are authored directly by members of the Cochrane Collaboration, developed using rigorous standards to identify, appraise, and synthesize the most scientifically valid evidence to answer specific research questions in all areas of healthcare and administration (About Cochrane Reviews, n.d.). Producing reviews with reduced bias and increased transparency is a key aspect of the Cochrane model.

The Joanna Briggs Institute

The Joanna Briggs Institute (JBI) works to connect nurses and other healthcare professionals to EBP resources, to improve patient outcomes, and to ensure the provision of high-quality care across a wide range of specialties (Joanna Briggs Insititute EBP resources, n.d.). The JBI Evidence-Based Database provides access to JBI-authored systematic reviews and evidence summaries via the Ovid platform.

UpToDate

UpToDate is a well-known, easy-to-navigate point-of-care electronic resource that includes over 11,000 physician-authored topic reviews addressing multiple clinical questions, covering 25 medical specialties (About Us – UpToDate, n.d.). A 2012 study by Isaac et al. found that provider use of UpToDate was associated with slightly reduced length of stay and lower mortality rates (Isaac et al., 2012).

DynaMed

DynaMed also provides evidence summaries on a variety of clinical topics. DynaMed applies Level of Evidence ratings (ranging from Level 1 to Level 3) to evidence summaries using a systematic process. This rating system makes it easy for users to quickly understand the quality of summarized evidence, as well as the primary rationale behind the rating. (What We Publish | DynaMed, n.d.). Additionally, when compared to other evidence summary databases, DynaMed was found to update its content most often (Banzi et al., 2011).

Hybrid Databases

Trip and Google Scholar are *hybrid databases*, which provide access to both primary and secondary sources of information.

Trip

Trip searches multiple levels of clinically focused evidence, offering researcher access to primary research via integration with Medline/PubMed as well as secondary research through integration with Cochrane and professional organizations' published clinicals guidelines (among other sources; Sources searched by Trip – Trip Database Blog, n.d.). A unique feature of Trip is that it organizes results by evidence type, allowing users to select particular categories most relevant to their particular needs. Categories include evidence-based synopses, systematic reviews, guidelines, and primary research (Fyfe, 2007; Sources searched by Trip – Trip Database Blog, n.d.). While basic searching of Trip is free, a subscription is required to access certain additional search features and full-text results.

Google Scholar

Google Scholar offers a robust, intuitive, and free database, covering a wide variety of academic disciplines, pulling its information from numerous sources. Although omnipresent, concerns with search algorithm transparency, quality of indexed content, and lack of advanced searching features keep Google Scholar from being considered an essential biomedical database for research development (Haddaway et al., 2015). However, it has been shown to be a good source for grey literature acquisition (conference proceedings/abstracts, institutional repository content, white papers, etc.), an especially important component when developing searches in support of systematic reviews and meta-analyses (Haddaway et al., 2015). Similarly, evidence has shown that Google Scholar may provide more relevant results for quick clinical questions as well as more comprehensive results overall, but at the cost of worse precision (more "noise") when compared to PubMed (Nourbakhsh et al., 2012; Shariff et al., 2013).

Table 3.1 | Commonly Used Databases

Database	Website	Description	Cost
Medline (PubMed)	https://www.ncbi.nlm.nih.gov/pubmed	PubMed features more than 30 million citations for biomedical literature from Medline, life science journals, and online books. Citations may include links to full-text content from PubMed Central and publisher websites.	Free

Table 3.1 | Commonly Used Databases

Medline (Ovid)	https://www.ovid.com/product-details.901.html	Medline via the Ovid platform provides searchers with seamless and up-to-the-minute access to over 23 million of the latest bibliographic citations and author abstracts from more than 5,600 biomedicine and life sciences journals in nearly 40 languages.	Subscription
Cumulative Index to Nursing and Allied Health Literature (CINAHL)	https://www.ebscohost.com/nursing/products/cinahl-databases	CINAHL provides indexing of top nursing and allied health literature, including nursing journals and publications from the National League for Nursing and the American Nurses Association. Nearly 5,500 journals are indexed covering a wide range of topics including nursing, biomedicine, health sciences librarianship, alternative/complementary medicine, consumer health, and 17 allied health disciplines.	Subscription
PsycINFO	https://www.apa.org/pubs/databases/psycinfo/	PsycINFO is a database of abstracts of literature in the fields of psychology and mental health. It is produced by the American Psychological Association and indexes nearly 2,500 behavioral and social sciences journals, 99% of which are peer-reviewed.	Subscription
Education Resources Information Center (ERIC)	https://eric.ed.gov	ERIC is an online digital library of education research and information, providing access to 1.5 million citations of journal articles and other education-related materials.	Free
EMBASE	https://www.embase.com	EMBASE is a biomedical and pharmacological bibliographic database with 37.2 million+ records from almost 8,100 currently published journals, a portion of which are not available in Medline.	Subscription

continues

Table 3.1 | Commonly Used Databases *(cont.)*

Cochrane Library	https://www.cochranelibrary.com	The Cochrane Library is a collection of databases that contain different types of high-quality, independent evidence to inform healthcare decision-making, including the Cochrane Database of Systematic Reviews, a leading resource for systematic reviews in healthcare.	Subscription
Joanna Briggs Institute Evidence-Based Database (Ovid)	http://know.lww.com/JBI-resources.html	This site features evidence-based content and tools from the Joanna Briggs Institute, summarizing research in easy to locate, understand, and distribute formats, with a focus on nursing's needs. Summarizes the best available evidence to improve patient outcomes through tailored clinical practice guidelines.	Subscription
UpToDate	https://www.uptodate.com/	UpToDate is an evidence-based clinical resource that includes medical and patient information, access to Lexi-comp drug monographs and drug-to-drug interactions, and medical calculators. UpToDate is written by over 7,100 physician authors, editors, and peer reviewers.	Subscription
DynaMed	https://www.dynamed.com	DynaMed is an evidence-based, clinical decision support tool that combines the most current clinical evidence with guidance from leading experts in a user-friendly, personalized experience.	Subscription
Trip	http://www.tripdatabase.com	Trip is a clinical search engine designed to allow users to quickly and easily find and use high-quality research evidence to support their practice and care.	Free*
Google Scholar	https://scholar.google.com	Google Scholar is a freely accessible web search engine that indexes the full text or metadata of scholarly literature across a wide variety of academic disciplines.	Free

*No cost for basic use, with limited access and features. Fees charged for more robust features.

The Nuts and Bolts of Literature Searching

Although databases may have different scopes, contents, and layouts, many employ similar search mechanics. With the exceptions of DynaMed, UptoDate, and Google Scholar, most databases feature options for basic as well as more advanced searching. Many use controlled vocabularies; support Boolean operators, truncation and wildcard symbols, explode and focus features, limits, and filters; and offer multiple methods to save and export both searches and search results. Within this section, we explore these details of database searching. Illustrative examples from PubMed, Ovid Medline, and CINAHL are provided throughout.

Basic and Advanced Searching

Basic searching refers to simple searches, typically limited to one or two concepts. While Boolean operators (AND, OR, NOT) may be used in basic searches, they are typically not extensively relied upon in this mode of searching. Basic searching may be used to gather background data or to take a quick initial look into the literature. In PubMed, the default method of searching is via the basic search bar, prominently displayed upon navigating to PubMed, shown in Figure 3.1. However, by clicking on the "Advanced" search feature on the bottom-left side of the search bar, users can navigate to an alternative PubMed search page.

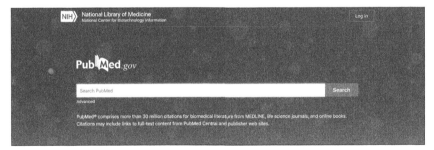

Figure 3.1 | PubMed homepage. Basic search bar featured and "Advanced" link just below it.

The PubMed advanced search page, shown in Figure 3.2, contains a search builder that allows for the construction of more nuanced searches. When developing advanced searches, it is best to search each concept of your question separately. Earlier in this chapter we discussed PICO questions, specifically using the concepts identified within our PICO questions to help establish initial search terms. From those terms identified earlier in this chapter, we will search for the most important concepts of *congestive heart failure*, *health literacy*, and *mortality*. Each term will be searched in PubMed individually. The advanced search builder will help us combine each term easily after each is searched. See Figures 3.2, 3.3, 3.4, and 3.5 for a visual overview of this portion of the search building process.

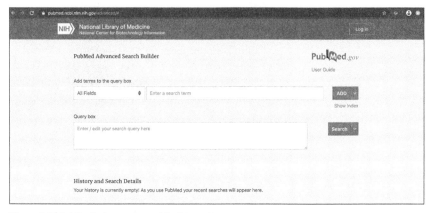

Figure 3.2 | PubMed advanced search builder webpage.

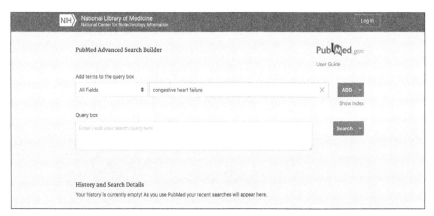

Figure 3.3 | Enter your first term in the "Add terms to the query box." After entering "congestive heart failure," click the "Add" button (to right of the "Search" box). This will move the term into the "Query" box below.

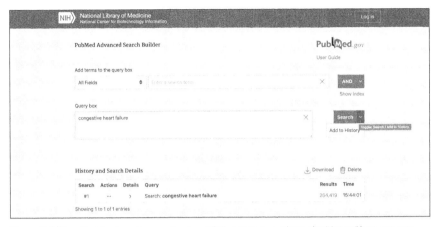

Figure 3.4 | Now that the term "congestive heart failure" has moved into the "Query" box, you can click on the downward white arrow just to the right of the blue "Search" box. This will open up an option to "Add to History" Click this because it will allow you to move the search term directly into the "History and Search Details" section at the bottom of the page. Once there, you can continue to build the advanced search.

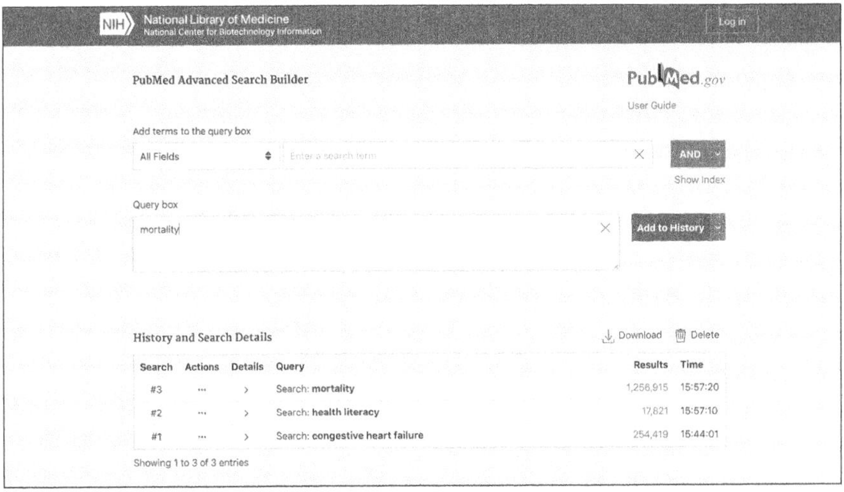

Figure 3.5 | Search any remaining terms in the same fashion as above. You will see that once you use the "Add to History" feature, the blue box will change and default to that option. Once all terms have been imported into the PubMed "History and Search Details" bar, you are ready to bring these terms together and search them.

Boolean Operators

Once all terms are seen in PubMed's "History and Search Details," Boolean operators are systematically applied. The ability to combine discrete terms using Boolean operators 'AND', 'OR', 'NOT' is one of the hallmarks of advanced searching and allows for the creation of robust searches with more focused results. The Boolean operator 'AND' is used to join terms, so that multiple concepts can be searched at the same time. Any returned citations will encompass all the terms searched. Using the example PICO concepts, the search "congestive heart failure AND health literacy AND mortality" would be used to locate articles that contain each concept. In this manner, 'AND' serves as a means to reduce the amount of literature returned, while ensuring the results remain pertinent.

In some scenarios, the term 'OR' might be applied to search terms. The use of 'OR' will expand results, identifying references that use any one of the terms linked by 'OR'. In our PICO example, we might find that limiting the search to my initially defined outcome of "mortality" too constraining, resulting in fewer articles being found than anticipated. We could instead search "mortality OR morbidity" to effectively expand the search. Typically, researchers use the Boolean operator 'OR' to link synonyms, or closely aligned terms.

Finally, there is also the option of using the 'NOT' to combine search terms. 'NOT' will exclude all terms that follow it from the returned data set. Caution is advised, however, as 'NOT' is a very powerful Boolean operator. As such, it should be used sparingly. For example, when looking at congestive heart failure, a researcher might be tempted to refine results using the search "congestive heart failure NOT myocardial infarction." While doing so would indeed eliminate citations on "myocardial infarction" from returned results, it would also eliminate any congestive heart failure citations that simply mentioned the term "myocardial infarction." As such, 'NOT' should be used only after extensive searching has taken place. Once a researcher has a good sense of the type of literature being retuned, 'NOT' may be applied as a specific technique to more easily identify obscure or less common data.

Returning to our PubMed search in Figure 3.5, with key terms now in the "History and Search Details" box, it is time to combine our concepts with the Boolean operator 'AND.' Figures 3.6, 3.7, and 3.8 illustrate how we add each of our three concepts to the advanced search "Query" box. Once all terms are added, press the blue "Search" button to retrieve the results. Before we move on to analyze and refine these results, though, let's shift to another technique one might use to locate appropriate references: search fields and controlled vocabulary.

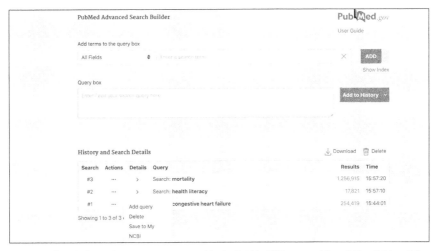

Figure 3.6 | With all initial concepts represented in the PubMed "History and Search Details" box, it is time to combine terms with the Boolean operator "AND." Look for the three dots under the "Actions" heading, to the left any term you want to combine. Choose the option to "Add query." In this case we have selected "congestive heart failure" and will add it to the "Query" box.

Figure 3.7 | When clicking on the three dots under the "Actions" heading next to "health literacy," you will see that the options from the drop-down menu have changed to include Boolean operators. As you want to build a search that will return literature that contains all of your search concepts, select the "Add with AND" from this menu. Do the same for each additional search term you wish to add to your search.

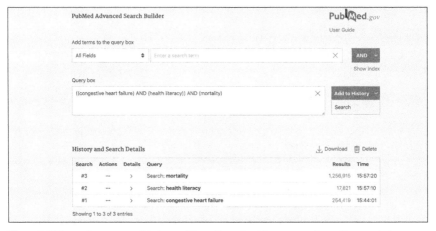

Figure 3.8 | Once all terms are added, your "Query" box should appear as above. Once again hover over the white arrow to the right of the "Add to History" to display the "Search" option. Click "Search" to run your search.

Search Fields and Controlled Vocabulary

Literature databases organize their content into various searchable fields. This technique allows for researchers to search for results not only by particular subjects of interest, but also by "Author," "Title," "Journal," "Affiliation," and many other fields. In Figure 3.6, notice the "All Fields" drop-down box in PubMed. This is where you can adjust your search, from the default of all searchable fields to one specific field, such as "Journal."

One of the most useful features of many literature databases are controlled vocabularies or subject headings. *Controlled vocabularies* organize topics in hierarchical fashion, or taxonomies, while also defining terms and identifying appropriate synonyms. The goal of controlled vocabularies is to provide searchers with greater levels of discovery than traditional keyword searching, as controlled vocabularies enable searching beyond data presented in title and abstract fields (where keyword searches typically search for information; Baumann, 2016). For example, when searching "chickenpox" in a database using controlled vocabulary, not only would my search return results on "chickenpox" but also on the alternate spelling "chicken pox" and the synonym "varicella." If searching using keyword searching only, searchers would need to type all three variations to achieve the same results.

Perhaps the best-known example of controlled vocabulary is Medline's Medical Subject Headings (MeSH). MeSH is a continuously evolving taxonomy, overseen by the NLM, that currently features over 25,000 terms (Spurlock, 2019). Specially trained indexers at NLM evaluate each article indexed in Medline and assign the most appropriate, descriptive MeSH terms available. As new terms and concepts arise in the published literature, MeSH is updated accordingly. CINHAL also uses controlled vocabulary, known as CINAHL Subject Headings. Other databases such as EMBASE and PyscINFO also have their own unique controlled vocabulary.

Using controlled vocabulary searching varies widely according to databases. In PubMed, MeSH searching is automatic. When a search is run, the database will seamlessly search for the most appropriate MeSH term available. At the same time, PubMed will search your term as a keyword.

If interested, you can see what PubMed is searching automatically. On the advanced search page, after terms have been loaded into the "History and Search Details," look for the "Details" column next to the term or search you are interested in. Click the "Details" arrow that corresponds to the term you are interested in to view what terms PubMed is actually searching (see Figure 3.9). When searching "congestive heart failure," for instance, the "Details" option shows us that PubMed mapped my original search term to the MeSH term *Heart Failure*, as well as several affiliated keywords.

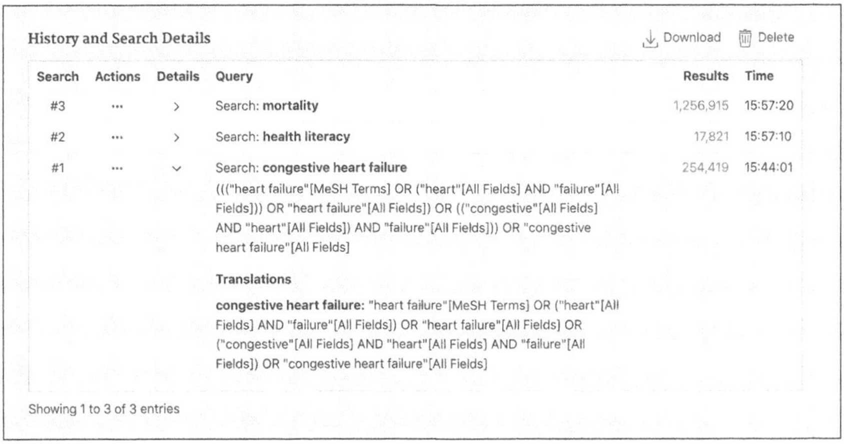
History and Search Details — Download — Delete

Search	Actions	Details	Query	Results	Time
#3	...	>	Search: **mortality**	1,256,915	15:57:20
#2	...	>	Search: **health literacy**	17,821	15:57:10
#1	...	⌄	Search: **congestive heart failure** ((("heart failure"[MeSH Terms] OR ("heart"[All Fields] AND "failure"[All Fields])) OR "heart failure"[All Fields]) OR (("congestive"[All Fields] AND "heart"[All Fields]) AND "failure"[All Fields])) OR "congestive heart failure"[All Fields] **Translations** **congestive heart failure:** "heart failure"[MeSH Terms] OR ("heart"[All Fields] AND "failure"[All Fields]) OR "heart failure"[All Fields] OR ("congestive"[All Fields] AND "heart"[All Fields] AND "failure"[All Fields]) OR "congestive heart failure"[All Fields]	254,419	15:44:01

Showing 1 to 3 of 3 entries

Figure 3.9 | The PubMed "Details" information, obtained by clicking on the arrow in the "Details" column to the left of the term or search of interest.

While PubMed applies MeSH headings automatically, behind the scenes, other databases utilize controlled vocabularies differently. Indeed, one of the key differences between PubMed and Ovid Medline is their differing approach to the use of MeSH. Within Ovid Medline, MeSH is front and center. When searching individual terms via this database, Ovid's default search will display a series of suggested MeSH headings. Instead of automatically choosing a MeSH heading for the user, Ovid prompts researchers to select their own MeSH heading from the returned list (see Figures 3.10 and 3.11). In this way, researchers are given more control over the search, ensuring returned results are more closely aligned to indented topics. In Figure 3.11, notice the MeSH term "Heart Failure" is recommended. This is the same MeSH heading PubMed automatically selected for us, as evidenced in the "Search details" box in Figure 3.8. When using Ovid Medline, the scope note (the circular "i" icon) to the extreme right of each MeSH term can be clicked to see the definition of the particular MeSH term selected. This is a good way to ensure the heading you have chosen indeed aligns with your intended topic.

Notice also in Figure 3.11, just under the blue underlined MeSH term "Heart Failure," there is a line that reflects exactly the original verbiage entered into the search box, as seen in Figure 3.10. If the user selects this bar to search, Ovid Medline will only search the term as a keyword. This means no MeSH headings will be applied to our search. Why might a researcher choose to search only keywords? The most common reason is to ensure that the most recent literature on a particular topic is discovered. Because MeSH headings take several months to be assigned to articles, searching by keyword helps return the most recent literature but at the expense of losing the utility provided by controlled vocabularies. Concerned users can direct Ovid Medline to search MeSH headings and the specified keyword by simply checking all boxes of interest prior to clicking the "Continue" button.

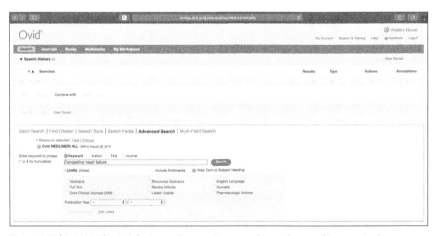

Figure 3.10 | Ovid Medline's default search page. Our example search term of "congestive heart failure" is entered into the search box. Clicking the blue "Search" button will begin the search. Notice below and to the right of the search bar the box next to "Map Term to Subject Heading" is checked. This is checked by default in Ovid databases.

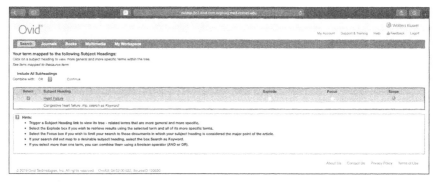

Figure 3.11 | Instead of automatically running the search (and mapping to a particular MeSH heading), Ovid Medline will bring you immediately to any potential MeSH headings it believes may be appropriate. Check those that are of interest and press "Continue."

Unlike PubMed and Ovid Medline, using the controlled vocabulary feature in CI-NAHL requires an extra step. However, it is quite easy to locate and search using CINAHL's Subject Headings if desired. Figure 3.12 shows CINAHL's default search page, on the EBSCO platform. Notice the "Suggest Subject Terms" box checked above the search term "congestive heart failure." This box must be manually selected by CINAHL users to search using controlled vocabulary. Once selected and searched, Figure 3.13 shows the various subject headings CINAHL suggests.

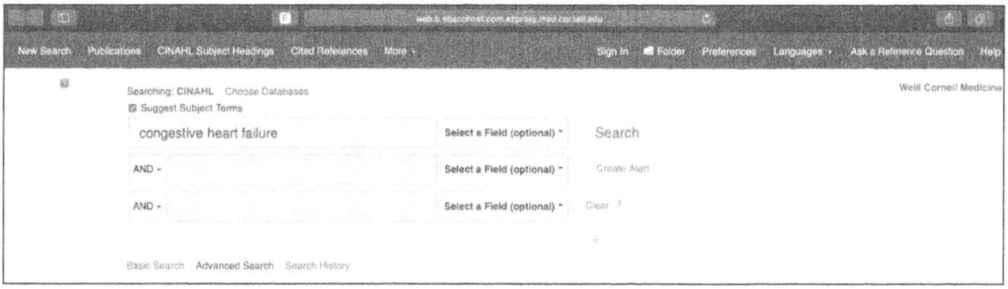

Figure 3.12 | When searching CINAHL via the EBSCO platform, the "Suggest Subject Terms" will not be automatically checked as in Ovid Medline. Click this box to access searching via CINAHL's controlled vocabulary.

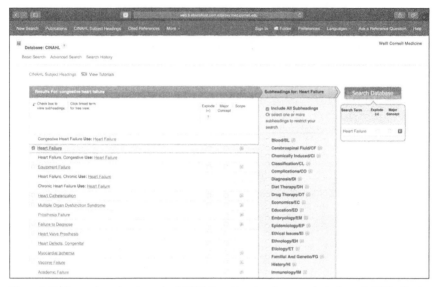

Figure 3.13 | Once selected and searched, CINAHL's subject heading page is similar to Ovid Medline's. Select the most appropriate term by checking the affiliated box to the left of the term.

Explode and Focus

Another important aspect of controlled vocabularies is the ability to further manage results using "Explode" or "Focus" (or "Major Concept") features. The hierarchical structure of controlled vocabularies allows for the use of "Explode." Notice in Ovid Medline (Figure 3.11) and CINAHL (Figure 3.13) the "Explode" column and checkbox to the right of the displayed subject headings. Checking these boxes will instruct the database to return not only all citations featuring the selected subject heading but also any more specific headings that fall below the selected term in the database's taxonomy. For instance, as seen in Figure 3.14, checking "Explode" in Ovid Medline would return not only results on *Heart Failure* but also those on *Cardio-Renal Syndrome, Paroxysmal Dyspnea, Cardiac Edema, Diastolic Heart Failure*, and *Systolic Heart Failure.* To learn what particular subject headings fall beneath the terms Ovid Medline or CINAHL suggest, simply click on the subject heading itself. Clicking on the words "Heart Failure" in Figure 3.11 will bring you to the subject tree displayed in Figure 3.14.

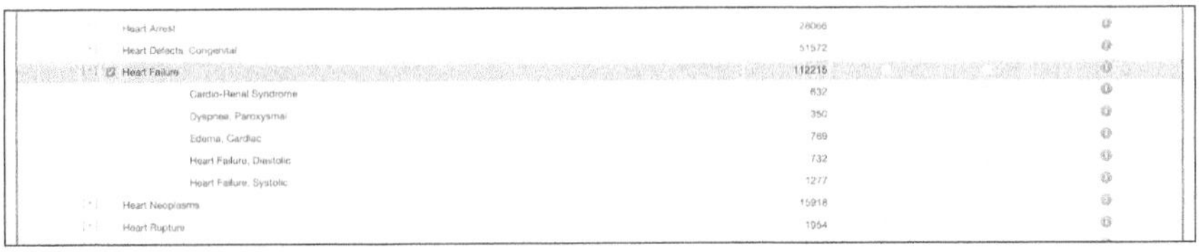

Figure 3.14 | Example in Ovid Medline of MeSH term *Heart Failure*, along with the specific terms that fall under it in the MeSH hierarchy.

Checking the "Explode" box will add each of these terms to the search, returning more results.

Whereas "Explode" serves to bring back more results, "Focus" (known as "Major Concept" in PubMed and CINAHL) tends to narrow results. When indexers evaluate articles to assign appropriate controlled vocabulary, they also identify the main points of each article. The most important concepts are noted and defined as the article's "Focus" or "Major Concept." Thus, researchers interested in articles with discrete, focused data can select the appropriate boxes to ensure that retuned articles more closely align to their desired concept.

Truncation

Truncation provides an additional method for database searching. This more advanced technique can be especially helpful when a search built with keywords or subject headings fails to return the results expected. Truncation allows for searching multiple roots or stems of terms. For example, in PubMed, Ovid Medline, and CINHAL, inserting an asterisk (*) at the end of the word stem will return multiple terms that contain the searched stem. Figure 3.15 highlights the terms searched in PubMed when using the truncated term "health liter*". Notice in Figure 3.15's search, however, that the MeSH term of "health literacy" was not applied by PubMed. Use of truncation (or other similar advanced methods, such as wildcard and adjacency searching) limits the usage of controlled vocabulary. That's not to say, however, that a search cannot contain both. Invested researchers can simply search truncated terms and controlled vocabulary separately and then use the Boolean operator 'OR' to combine all results. The final results of this larger search would then return results that were pulled by either truncated or controlled vocabulary terms.

| History and Search Details | | | | ⤓ Download | 🗑 Delete | |
Search	Actions	Details	Query		Results	Time
#5	...	∨	Search: **health liter***		247,230	17:15:48
			((((("health"[MeSH Terms] OR "health"[All Fields]) OR "health s"[All Fields]) OR "healthful"[All Fields]) OR "healthfulness"[All Fields]) OR "healths"[All Fields]) AND "liter*"[All Fields]			
			Translations			
			health: "health"[MeSH Terms] OR "health"[All Fields] OR "health's"[All Fields] OR "healthful"[All Fields] OR "healthfulness"[All Fields] OR "healths"[All Fields]			
#3	...	>	Search: **mortality**		1,256,915	15:57:20
#2	...	>	Search: **health literacy**		17,821	15:57:10
#1	...	>	Search: **congestive heart failure**		254,419	15:44:01

Showing 1 to 4 of 4 entries

Figure 3.15 | Viewing the "Details" in PubMed shows the exact terms a truncated search has included among returned results. Here is what was searched when "health liter*" was entered.

Next Steps—Search Results

After executing your search, it is time to examine the results. Even though a preliminary search has been run, quality literature searches are often an iterative process. Do not get discouraged if your first search does not appear as fruitful as expected. Retrieved results may be more numerous or less relevant than anticipated.

Filters and limits help further refine results. Typically, these can be found in the left-hand column of search result pages. Filters and limits are applied to narrow retrieved results, eliminating results that do not meet the defined criteria. For instance, in PubMed, a searcher may limit retuned results by *Age group, Article type, Publication date, Language,* and *Sex.* For example, in Figure 3.16, we selected to filter by *Publication date,* specifically articles published between 2015 and 2020. This reduced the results of our example PICO-derived search from 45 to 24 citations.

PubMed also gives the option to "clear" assigned filters. At times, filters applied may end up being too limiting. If this occurs, simply clear the applied filters to bring back the original, unfiltered set of results.

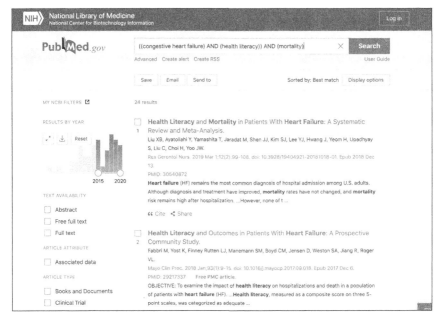

Figure 3.16 | Filters available can be seen in the left-hand column of PubMed's search results. Click the particular filter to apply it to the citations shown in the main column. Here, using the bar graph to the left of the first citation has been used to filter by publication date, allowing for only articles published between 2015 and 2020 to appear in the results. Scroll down and click on "Additional filters" (not shown here) at the bottom of the left-hand column to explore other filters available, such as *Age*, *Language*, and *Sex*.

Returned results may also be fewer than anticipated or seem a bit off-topic. In these cases, take a close look at the citations available. Open those most relevant to your topic of interest. The abstract page can often help locate additional articles in multiple ways. For instance, in Figure 3.17, look to the column to the right of the abstract. Here you will find two useful features: "Similar articles" and "Cited by..." Either click on these or simply scroll down the abstract page to identify citations of similar scope or content.

Additionally, clicking on the "MeSH terms" to the right or scrolling down the abstract page will bring searchers each of the MeSH headings that have been assigned to this abstract. Figure 3.18 shows the MeSH headings applied to the citation selected in Figure 3.17 for the article titled "Health Literacy Mediates the Relationship Between Age and Health Outcomes in Patients With Heart Failure." Closely evaluate these terms to locate other subject headings or concepts that may help expand, or better yet, capture your subject of interest. For example, in Figure 3.18, the MeSH headings of *Health Knowledge, Attitudes, Practice,* and *Treatment Outcome* may be useful concepts to expand the results generated by our example PICO search.

To search identified MeSH terms of interest, simply click on the desired MeSH heading. This will allow you to search the term and ultimately integrate it into PubMed's "History and Search Details" so that you can continue to build your advanced search. One thing to keep in mind with this particular strategy: MeSH headings are not applied automatically to MEDLINE citations but rather are added by indexers manually. When apprising newer articles, MeSH headings may not have yet been applied; thus, this particular strategy will not be valid.

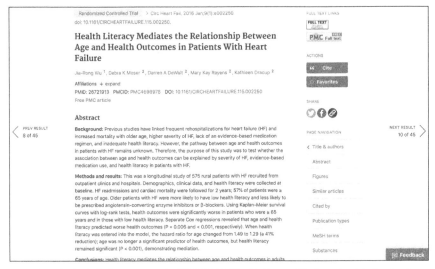

Figure 3.17 | PubMed's abstract record of Wu's [2016] "Health Literacy Mediates the Relationship Between Age and Health Outcomes in Patients With Heart Failure." See the "Similar articles" and "Cited by" features in the right-hand column for additional articles that may also be of interest.

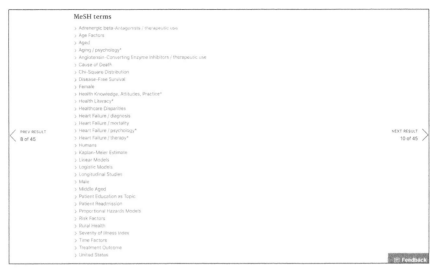

Figure 3.18 | PubMed's abstract record of MeSH terms applied to Wu's [2016] "Health Literacy Mediates the Relationship Between Age and Health Outcomes in Patients With Heart Failure." Clicking any of these subject headings will allow the user to search that term.

Once you are content with search results, it is time to save and export your findings. Each database has its own particular methods and tools established to assist with this process. PubMed, for instance, allows you to send results to your email, citation managers, or a "Clipboard." Refer to Figure 3.16 and note the boxes "Save," "Email," and "Send to" just under the search bar. PubMed's Clipboard is a space where you can group particular citations of interest pulled from multiple searches. Saving searches is accomplished through establishing a free NCBI account (NCBI Sign In Page, n.d.). An NCBI account also allows for the creation of auto alerts, which enable the results of predefined searches to be sent to a designated email address at specific intervals. See Figure 3.16, top-right corner where the button "Log in" appears. Click this to sign up and into your NCBI account. In Ovid Medline, important citations can be grouped together via the "Keep Selected" option. Citations can also be saved as PDFs, imported into citation management software, emailed, and more. Searches can be saved, and alerts created, in Ovid's MyWorkspace. CINAHL provides a "Folder" to organize your selected citations. Select and place all citations of relevance in this folder. From here, the contents then can be printed, emailed, or exported to a citation manager. MyEBSCOhost allows for the search saving and creation of CINHAL-generated alerts.

Management of Evidence Retrieved

As literature is identified, it is important to organize your citations and articles. Tables of evidence and citation management software offer two approaches that help with the process of data organization and sharing.

Tables of Evidence

Tables of evidence are constructed from the most pertinent articles located during the literature search process. Important attributes of retrieved articles are recorded in Microsoft Excel or Google Sheets files. Data collected should be customized to the specific project of interest (EBP, QI, or research) and may include:

Author and Year; Article Title; Source (journal title, volume and issue); Database; Study Design/Methods; Theoretical Framework, Setting (target population, geographic location, facility type, providers, etc.); Study Sample; Outcome Measures (may include validity and reliability); Quality of Evidence; Findings/Results; Limitations; Gaps; Relevance of Data to Research Question (see Table 3.2).

Table 3.2 | Example Table of Evidence

Authors, Year	Study Design	Sample	Outcome Measure	Results	Relevance to Question
Mayberry, L. S., Schildcrout, J. S., et al., 2018	5-year prospective cohort study; designed to examine how health literacy affects care transitions and outcomes.	N = 3000 patients treated at Vanderbilt University Hospital October 11, 2011 through December 18, 2015.	Mortality; gathered from the Social Security Administration's Death Master File (DMF), documentation in the electronic health record, family report, and obituaries.	Lower health literacy levels were associated with a higher probability of 1-year mortality in the base model (total effect AOR=1.31, CI [1.01, 1.69]).	Health literacy was indirectly associated with 1-year mortality among adults with cardiovascular disease.

Table 3.2 | Example Table of Evidence

Candace D. McNaughton, MD, MPH, Courtney Cawthon, MPH, et al., 2015	Retrospective cohort study	N = 1379 patients, average age was 63.1 years, 566 (41.0%) were female, and 324 (23.5%) had low health literacy.	Primary outcome was all-cause mortality. Secondary outcomes included rehospitalization, time to first emergency department visit within 90 days of discharge.		Lower health literacy was associated with increased risk of death after hospitalization for acute heart failure.

After establishing the data points of relevance to your research question, begin looking at the articles you have identified. Much of the information necessary for your table of evidence will be available within the abstracts of your selected articles. Because article abstracts are easily located at the beginning of articles, they can provide a quick source of important data. As you complete your tables, keep in mind the goal is to summarize article content and determine applicability to the research question of interest (Bernhofer, 2015). Another point to consider: Evidence tables are also used during data synthesis and should be considered an important, early step of the *A: Appraisal of Evidence* portion of the PEACE model (Phillippi et al., 2016; Tahan et al., 2016).

Citation Managers

Citation managers offer another way to organize and manage the results of literature reviews. Citations generated from the databases searched can be imported into programs such as Endnote, Sciwheel (formerly F1000 Workspace), and Mendeley (see Table 3.3). Once in a citation manager, PDFs can be attached and annotated, collections can be shared, and bibliographies can be easily created. Many of these electronic reference management resources are integrated with Microsoft Word and Google Docs. This integration enables citations from an Endnote project folder, for example, to be imported into a paper being developed. Authors can then cite as they write, placing in-text citations in their proper place in the text and formatting bibliographies in whichever desired citation style or journal format is selected (APA, Chicago, JAMA, etc.; Robb & Shellenbarger, 2014). The features and cost of each citation manager differ, so take some time to evaluate your options. Does your affiliated hospital or university library provide access to citation management software? Which ones do your colleagues and collaborators use? Which features are important to you? Like selecting which databases to search, selecting citation management software can be a daunting process. Discussing your questions and needs with more seasoned nurse researchers or a librarian is perfectly acceptable.

Table 3.3 | Common Citation Management Software

Citation Manage- ment Software	Website	Features	Cost
Endnote Desktop	https://endnote. com/	Cite references in Microsoft Word 7,000+ predefined citation styles available, plus create your own One-click find full-text option Unlimited reference and file attachment storage	Subscription
Endnote Online	https://access. clarivate.com/ login?app= endnote	Access library from anywhere Cite references in Microsoft Word Top 21 most commonly used citation styles available 50,000 max reference and 2 GB max of file attachment storage	Free*
Sciwheel (formerly F1000 Workspace)	https://sciwheel. com/	Access library from anywhere Instantly save references from the web Highlight and annotate PDFs and web pages Find and cite references in Microsoft Word and Google Docs Multiple citation styles, with ability to add your own Easy collaboration with coauthors	Free*
Mendeley	https://www. mendeley.com	Access library from anywhere Ability to annotate PDFs Cite references in Microsoft Word Multiple citation styles, with ability to add your own	Free

*No cost for basic use, with limited access and features. Fees charged for more robust features.

Summary

Literature searching is an important part of any project. The information presented in this chapter is only a portion of the various approaches to evidence retrieval used by researchers. Allot plenty of time to work through this process. Find the databases, search methods, and citation management software that work best for you. Before moving on to the next chapter, consider the following takeaway points:

- Take time to evaluate the various databases available to you. Select and search those databases most relevant to your particular topic of interest. Search multiple databases to ensure a wide breadth of results.

- Use all the features of databases to construct quality searches. Experiment with Boolean operators, controlled vocabulary, keywords, truncation, and limits; see which combinations return the best evidence.

- Develop a table of evidence to help organize and analyze your findings.

- Consider using citation management software to help organize citations and greatly assist when writing manuscripts.

- Don't hesitate to consult with nurse researchers or librarians. Their expertise can make your evidence review process more impactful and less stressful.

Review Questions

1. Databases such as UpToDate and DynaMed can best be used to support what type of projects/activities/studies?

   A. EBP projects

   B. QI activities

   C. Research studies

   D. None of the above

   Answer: A. Databases such as UpToDate and DynaMed can best support EBP projects because they provide comprehensive overviews of high-quality evidence on focused clinical topics.

2. PubMed and Ovid Medline both search the same database.

   A. True

   B. False

   Answer: A. True. PubMed and Ovid Medline are different digital platforms that each search the same medical database (Medline).

3. What are Medical Subject Headings (MeSH)?

    A. A diagnostic coding system of the World Health Organization created to classify various disease states.

    B. A library classification system developed by the National Library of Medicine meant to organize books and other published materials.

    C. A controlled vocabulary applied to articles in Medline that allows for the searching of synonyms and spelling variations.

    D. A biomedical database developed by the National Library of Medicine that cites over 25 million references.

Answer: C. MeSH or Medical Subject Headings help Medline identify and search synonyms and spelling variations.

4. Filters can be applied to literature search results. Filters can help to:

    A. Limit the number of search results

    B. Identify the most recent literature

    C. Find articles in Spanish

    D. All of the above

Answer: D. Filters can be applied to help focus your results in a variety of ways. They exist to help quickly eliminate results that may not be relevant.

5. Tables of evidence DO NOT typically include what type of information?

    A. Author

    B. Citation management software used

    C. Study sample/number of research subjects

    D. Quality appraisal of evidence

Answer: B. Tables of evidence do not need to mention citation management software information. Citation management software is chiefly used to help organize citations and formulate bibliographies while writing papers. This process typically occurs after data has been placed into a table of evidence.

References

About Cochrane Reviews. (n.d.). https://www.cochranelibrary.com/about/about-cochrane-reviews

About Us - UpToDate. (n.d.). https://www.uptodate.com/home/about-us

Agoritsas, T., Vandvik, P. O., Neumann, I., Rochwerg, B., Jaeschke, R., Hayward, R., ... McKibbon, K. A. (2015). Finding current best evidence. In G. Guyatt, D. Rennie, M. O. Meade, & D. J. Cook (Eds.), *Users' guides to the medical literature: A manual for evidence-based clinical practice* (3rd ed.). McGraw-Hill Education.

Banzi, R., Cinquini, M., Liberati, A., Moschetti, I., Pecoraro, V., Tagliabue, L., & Moja, L. (2011). Speed of updating online evidence based point of care summaries: Prospective cohort analysis. *BMJ (Clinical Research Ed.), 343*, d5856. doi:10.1136/bmj.d5856

Baumann, N. (2016). How to use the medical subject headings (MeSH). *International Journal of Clinical Practice, 70*(2), 171–174. https://doi.org/10.1111/ijcp.12767

Bernhofer, E. I. (2015). Reviewing the literature: Essential first step in research, quality improvement, and implementation of evidence-based practice. *Journal for Nurses in Professional Development, 31*(4), 191–196; quiz E1. doi:10.1097/NND.0000000000000171

Carman, M. J., Wolf, L. A., Henderson, D., Kamienski, M., Koziol-McLain, J., Manton, A., & Moon, M. D. (2013). Developing your clinical question: The key to successful research. *Journal of Emergency Nursing, 39*(3), 299–301. doi:10.1016/j.jen.2013.01.011

CINAHL Database. (n.d.). EBSCO Health. https://health.ebsco.com/products/the-cinahl-database

Conner, B. (2014). Differentiating research, evidence-based practice, and quality improvement. *American Nurse Today, 9*(6).

Embase content (n.d.). https://www.elsevier.com/solutions/embase-biomedical-research/embase-coverage-and-content

ERIC content. (n.d.). https://eric.ed.gov/?faq-content

Eriksen, M. B., & Frandsen, T. F. (2018). The impact of patient, intervention, comparison, outcome (PICO) as a search strategy tool on literature search quality: A systematic review. *Journal of the Medical Library Association, 106*(4), 420–431. doi:10.5195/jmla.2018.345

Fyfe, T. (2007). Turning research into practice (TRIP). *Journal of the Medical Library Association, 95*(2), 215–216. doi:10.3163/1536-5050.95.2.215

Gerberi, D., & Shirk Marienau, M. (2017). Literature searching for practice research. *AANA Journal, 85*(3), 195–204.

Haddaway, N. R., Collins, A. M., Coughlin, D., & Kirk, S. (2015). The role of Google Scholar in evidence reviews and its applicability to grey literature searching. *PLOS One, 10*(9), e0138237. doi:10.1371/journal.pone.0138237

Ho, G. J., Liew, S. M., Ng, C. J., Hisham Shunmugam, R., & Glasziou, P. (2016). Development of a search strategy for an evidence based retrieval service. *PLOS One, 11*(12), e0167170. doi:10.1371/journal.pone.0167170

Isaac, T., Zheng, J., & Jha, A. (2012). Use of UpToDate and outcomes in US hospitals. *Journal of Hospital Medicine (Online), 7*(2), 85–90. doi:10.1002/jhm.944

Joanna Briggs Insititute EBP resources. (n.d.). http://know.lww.com/JBI-resources.html

NCBI Sign In Page. (n.d.). https://www.ncbi.nlm.nih.gov/account/?back_url=https%3A%2F%2Fwww.ncbi.nlm.nih.gov%2F

Nourbakhsh, E., Nugent, R., Wang, H., Cevik, C., & Nugent, K. (2012). Medical literature searches: A comparison of PubMed and Google Scholar. *Health Information and Libraries Journal, 29*(3), 214–222. https://doi.org/10.1111/j.1471-1842.2012.00992.x

Ovid MEDLINE. (n.d.). https://www.ovid.com/product-details.901.html

Phillippi, J., Hande, K., & Allison, T. L. (2016). The literature table as a prompt for careful appraisal. *The Journal of Nursing Education, 55*(10), 599–600. doi:10.3928/01484834-20160914-13

PsycINFO. (n.d.). https://www.apa.org/pubs/databases/psycinfo?tab=3

PubMed Clinical Queries. (n.d.). https://www.ncbi.nlm.nih.gov/pubmed/clinical

Robb, M., & Shellenbarger, T. (2014). Strategies for searching and managing evidence-based practice resources. *Journal of Continuing Education in Nursing, 45*(10), 461–466. doi:10.3928/00220124-20140916-01

Shariff, S. Z., Bejaimal, S. A., Sontrop, J. M., Iansavichus, A. V., Haynes, R. B., Weir, M. A., & Garg, A. X. (2013). Retrieving clinical evidence: A comparison of PubMed and Google Scholar for quick clinical searches. *Journal of Medical Internet Research, 15*(8), e164. doi:10.2196/jmir.2624

Sources searched by Trip – Trip Database Blog. (n.d.). https://blog.tripdatabase.com/2017/10/27/sources-searched-by-trip/

Spurlock, D. (2019). Searching the literature in preparation for research: Strategies that matter. *The Journal of Nursing Education, 58*(8), 441–443. doi:10.3928/01484834-20190719-02

Tahan, H. M., Rivera, R. R., Carter, E. J., Gallagher, K. A., Fitzpatrick, J. J., & Manzano, W. M. (2016). Evidence-based nursing practice: The PEACE framework. *Nurse Leader, 14*(1), 57–61. doi:10.1016/j.mnl.2015.07.012

U.S. National Library of Medicine. (n.d.). MEDLINE: Description of the database. https://www.nlm.nih.gov/bsd/medline.html

Web of Science. (n.d.). Web of Science Group. https://clarivate.com/webofsciencegroup/solutions/web-of-science/

Web of Science Group. (n.d.). Journal citation reports. https://clarivate.com/webofsciencegroup/solutions/journal-citation-reports/

What We Publish | DynaMed. (n.d.). https://www.dynamed.com/home/about/what-we-publish

PEACE MODEL

P | **PROBLEM IDENTIFICATION**
Formulate the clinical question (**PICO**):
- **P** | Patient Population
- **I** | Intervention
- **C** | Comparison of Intervention
- **O** | Outcome

E | **EVIDENCE REVIEW**
Review evidence relevant to your clinical question by searching databases.

A | **APPRAISE EVIDENCE**
Appraise the evidence that appears highest in the hierarchy of scientific evidence for its quality and applicability to practice.

C | **CHANGE PRACTICE OR CONDUCT RESEARCH**
If evidence is sufficient, embark on improvement project to address practice change.
If evidence is insufficient to warrant practice change, conduct research.

E | **EVALUATE AND DISSEMINATE FINDINGS**
Evaluate the impact of the implemented practice change and research results.
Disseminate findings through publication, oral, and poster presentations.

4

APPRAISE
THE EVIDENCE

–Carolyn Sun, PhD, RN, ANP-BC

KEYWORDS | PHRASES

evidence, appraisal, nursing research, quality improvement, quality appraisal, evidence-based practice

CHAPTER OBJECTIVES

After studying this chapter, learners will be able to:

1. Describe the importance of appraising evidence.
2. Identify an appropriate tool to evaluate a research study.
3. Appraise a research study and make conclusions about its strengths and weaknesses.

Introduction

Now that you have identified your problem (P), developed your PICO question, and done an evidence review (E), the next step is to begin A—appraise the evidence. In this chapter, the steps needed to assess and appraise the quality of evidence in a study are identified. Also, through a model of critiquing the literature, findings are examined to help determine whether the results of the study are valid and whether they can be applied to patient care or practice.

But before we begin the evidence appraisal, take a moment to think about why you need to appraise the quality of the evidence. We know that evidence changes over time, so even when we think we know the answer, it's important to critique research to determine its strengths and weaknesses (McMenamin et al., 2019). You might have heard the phrase, "All evidence is not created equally" or, "Published literature does not equal good quality literature." This is true! For an example to help you think this through, consider the following studies.

A Tale of Two Studies: Meditation and Hypertension Outcomes

Nurse Margaret wants to find out whether daily meditation can help reduce blood pressure (BP). Her PICO question is:

> **P**opulation: In adults with hypertension
>
> **I**ntervention: does meditation
>
> **C**omparison: compared to no meditation
>
> **O**utcome: result in reduced blood pressure?

Margaret picks five of her friends and family members with self-reported hypertension and measures their BP once in the morning, teaches them techniques for meditation, and then measures their BP one additional time on the same day of the intervention. She finds that all five have reduced BP in the second reading and concludes that meditation is an effective intervention to reduce BP.

Nurse Sarah has the same PICO question. She decides to conduct the study with a different approach. She recruits 100 patients with hypertension who do not currently practice meditation and conducts an informational survey that asks them about their race, gender, age, medications, current health issues, and dietary and exercise habits. She randomly divides them into two groups using a coin toss; one group of 50 is the control group; the remainder are the intervention group. For all the patients, she measures their BP twice, two minutes apart, daily for two weeks. Then she teaches the intervention group a meditation exercise. She asks them to practice the meditation every day for one month and keep a record of whether they completed the intervention each day. For both groups, she continues to measure their BP twice, two minutes apart every day at the same time as the preintervention phase throughout the month of the intervention. She continues to measure the BP in the same way for two weeks after the intervention phase finishes. Sarah conducts statistical analyses to account for demographic differences, medications, diagnoses, exercise, dietary habits, and the frequency that the participant recorded doing the intervention. Similar to Margaret, she finds a statistically significant improvement in the intervention group and concludes that meditation can improve BP.

While both groups determined that meditation has a beneficial effect on hypertension, Sarah's study is more sound. Can you think of all the reasons Margaret's study is flawed?

We know that BP may be higher in the morning (Wang et al., 2017), so remeasuring BP later on the same day could result in a decreased BP that has nothing to do with the intervention. Also, according to the American Heart Association guidelines, you must have at least two BP measurements on more than two occasions to diagnose hypertension (Whelton et al., 2018). Without these, Margaret cannot confirm the self-reported diagnoses of hypertension. Sarah solves these problems by measuring several times over several weeks, at the same time each day. She also considered things that could affect both the intervention and the outcome being measured, like other medical conditions, whether participants were already doing meditation, race, gender, and ethnicity. We also should consider the sample size to make sure that we have enough people to detect a difference between those who did the intervention and those who didn't (Charan & Biswas, 2013; Zodpey, 2004). We do not actually know if Sarah did a sample size calculation, but it is unlikely that Margaret had enough people in her sample to detect a difference before and after the intervention, even if there were no other confounding factors (e.g., the BP naturally going down after the morning reading).

All of these are just a few of the many things that should be considered when reviewing a study, but you can see right away that even studies that ask the same question vary widely in terms of quality. This brings us back to the point—we need to appraise the evidence so that we can determine the quality of the study. This helps us ascertain how meaningful the results are, or, in other words, the strength of the study's evidence. You may have seen Fineout-Overholt's pyramid of evidence (see Figure 4.1; Fineout-Overholt et al., 2010).

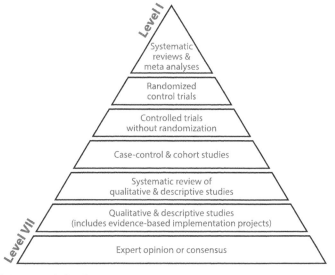

Figure 4.1 | The pyramid of evidence.

In Figure 4.1, you see that studies are rated as having different "levels" of evidence, with the strongest evidence being at the top of the pyramid (Level I) and the weakest evidence at the bottom (Level VII). According to the pyramid of evidence, different types of studies include characteristics that inherently make them higher or lower quality. For example, randomized controlled trials (like Sarah's) help to offset some biases by making sure that you don't select people you think are more likely to benefit from the intervention and put them into the intervention group by randomizing who gets the intervention. But how do you know which questions to ask? Where do you start?

There are four main steps to appraising the evidence (see Table 4.1).

Table 4.1 | Steps to Evaluate a Research Study

Step	Description
Step 1. Determine the type of study and appropriate tool to critique the study.	Because there are so many types of studies, it is important to choose an appropriate tool to ensure you are answering the right questions when reading a research study. Both the Joanna Briggs Institute and the Critical Appraisal Skills Programme have checklists for many types of studies.
Step 2: Read the article.	It is important to thoroughly read the article before you begin to appraise a study. As you read, bear in mind the authors' titles and affiliations and any conflicts of interest.
Step 3: Appraise the article.	Using the selected tool, appraise the article by answering the questions on the selected checklist. In our example, they are, briefly: 1. Inclusion/exclusion criteria. How were the participants selected? 2. Sample and setting. Who were the participants? Where was the study conducted? 3. Reliability and validity. Were instruments used valid (measuring the thing they intended to measure) and reliable (getting the same result each time)? 4. Measurement of the condition. Was the appropriate sample recruited? 5. and 6. Confounding. Could anything have biased the results? 7. Outcome measures. Were they measuring the thing they should measure to really capture the effect of the intervention? 8. Statistical analyses. Were the appropriate statistical tests conducted?

Table 4.1 | Steps to Evaluate a Research Study

Step 4. Summarize the results and make a decision.	Based on the results of your critique, decide whether you think the study is worth using as a basis for conducting further research or making a practice change.

Evidence Appraisal Example Using a Published Article

Gonzalez-Mercado and colleagues (2018) published a paper titled "The Health Related Quality of Life of Puerto Ricans During Cancer Treatments: A Pilot Study" in the *Puerto Rico Health Sciences Journal*. We will use this paper to demonstrate how to apply the critique process. The paper can be downloaded for free at https://www.ncbi.nlm.nih.gov/pmc/articles/PMC5863575/.

This is a study in which investigators examined the health-related quality of life (HRQOL) in Puerto Ricans undergoing cancer treatment. The authors used an existing survey instrument to measure HRQOL at one point in time in 79 adult cancer patients. They found that women had statistically significantly worse HRQOL compared to their male counterparts.

Step 1: Determine the Type of Study and Appropriate Tool to Critique the Study

The first step is to consider the type of article you are trying to appraise. This is important because you need to know which questions you should be asking. For example, if you are critiquing a cohort study, you would not need to ask whether the participants were properly randomized. Many published papers will tell you what kind of study you are reading in the title, but if not, you can often find the study type in the abstract or the methods section. In our example, you can see the type of study is included in the methods section of the abstract (see Figure 4.2; Gonzalez-Mercado et al., 2018).

The Health Related Quality of Life of Puerto Ricans during Cancer Treatments; a pilot study

Velda J. Gonzalez-Mercado, PhD, RN, Susan McMillan, PHD, ARNP, FAAN, Elsa Pedro, PharmD., Maribel Tirado-Gomez, MD, and Leorey N. Saligan, PhD, RN, CRNP, FAAN

· Author information · Copyright and License information Disclaimer

Abstract   Go to: ☑

Objective

To examine the health related quality of life (HRQOL) experienced by 79 Puerto Rican adults during cancer treatments.

Methods

This study used a descriptive, cross-sectional design. Participants completed a demographics form and the Functional Assessment of Cancer Therapy- General QOL questionnaire (FACT-G). Descriptive statistics were generated.

Results

Participants were ages 28–78; most of the participants had breast (38.0%), prostate (14.0%) and cervical and ovarian cancers (10.1%) treated with chemotherapy (45.6%). The participants had a mean total score on the FACT-G of 75.2 (SD = 18.9). As a group, the functional well-being was the most affected (mean 17.2, SD 6.8), and the Social/Familial was the least affected (mean 20.7, SD 6.0).

Conclusion

Cancer is the leading cause of death in the island of Puerto Rico. Female Puerto Rican cancer patients in this study sample had increased risk for experiencing worse: overall HRQOL, physical well-being and emotional well-being compared to males. Given that the Hispanic oncology population does not always report symptoms, risking under-assessment and under-management, this suggests there may be a greater need for HRQOL surveillance for this population.

Figure 4.2 | Example 1 abstract.

The abstract tells you that this is a descriptive, cross-sectional design. Now that you know which kind of study you have, you need to figure out the proper tool to use to critique the article. A useful table was published by Buccheri and Sharifi (2017) that we have adapted for use (see Table 4.2).

To use the table, look down the left-hand column for the type of study and follow across the row to see the different tools you could use to appraise the quality of that type of study. Many nursing studies are cross-sectional, like the one we are using for this example. (Remember that a *cross-sectional study* is a cross-section of a moment in time—this includes surveys that are only administered one time.) You can see there are two options listed in the table that you can choose for a cross-sectional study:

> *Joanna Briggs Institute. (2017). The Joanna Briggs Institute Critical Apprais-al tools for use in JBI Systematic Reviews: Checklist for Analytical Cross Sectional Studies. Available from: https://joannabriggs.org/sites/default/ files/2019-05/JBI_Critical_Appraisal-Checklist_for_Analytical_Cross_ Sectional_Studies2017_0.pdf*

Or

Downes, M. J., Brennan, M. L., Williams, H. C., & Dean, R. S. (2016). Development of a critical appraisal tool to assess the quality of cross-sectional studies (AXIS). BMJ Open, 6, e011458.

Both of these instruments are free to download (the final version of the AXIS tool is available here: https://bmjopen.bmj.com/content/bmjopen/6/12/e011458/DC2/embed/inline-supplementary-material-2.pdf?download=true). The AXIS tool is nice because very thorough explanations are given of what each of the terms mean, but the Joanna Briggs (JBI) tool is much shorter, which could make it a good choice if you have many papers to review. Essentially, the instruments ask the same questions, but the JBI tool has higher-level questions, and the AXIS tool has more detailed questions. For the purpose of this chapter we will use the Joanna Briggs tool, but you may want to refer to the AXIS tool for further explanations of certain terminology.

Step 2: Read the Article

Before beginning to critique the study, it is a good idea to read the article all the way through. You should already have some sense that the study you are critiquing fits the criteria you require for your study. That is to say, the purpose of the critique is to decide if the quality of the study is good enough to use as evidence going forward; it should not be to determine the topic of the study. Going back to our example of nurses Sarah and Margaret, they should have first reviewed what is already known about meditation as a means of lowering BP. After they have found several studies that are about the effects of meditation on BP, they should critique them. They may not have carefully read them at first when they were screening articles that could potentially help them decide whether the study was worth pursuing, but at this point, before beginning the critique they should take some time to carefully read the articles.

First, consider the title of the study. Confirm that this appears to be what you think you are looking for—occasionally, library links will send you to the wrong article, so you just want to double-check that everything sounds right. Many times you can determine the topic and the study design just from the title. Next, look at the authors and their credentials. As you read the study, this will help you decide whether the authors have sufficient expertise to conduct a study on this topic. For example, if you are reading a study about nursing work habits and all the authors are physicians, you may want to question why the authors did not bother to have an expert on the matter—in this instance, a nurse—as a coauthor on the study. A nurse may be able to help interpret what the results mean in a more meaningful way. Conversely,

Table 4.2 │ Tools for Evaluating Evidence

Name of Checklist/ Type of Evidence	Agree II (Brouwers et al., 2010)	CASP Checklist (CASP, 2017)	Cochrane Risk of Bias Tool (Higgins, Savović, Page, Elbers, & Sterne, 2019)	EPQA Guidelines (Lee, Johnson, Newhouse, & Warren, 2013)
Meta-analysis				
Systematic review		X		
Literature review				
Randomized controlled trial		X	X	
Cohort study		X		
Case-control study		X		
Meta-synthesis				
Qualitative study		X		
Expert opinion				
Evidence-based practice project				X
Quality improvement project				
Clinical practice guideline	X	X		
Cross-sectional study				

Adapted from Buccheri and Sharifi (2017)

	GRADE (Dijkers, 2013)	JBI Checklists (Joanna Briggs Institute, 2019)	Johns Hopkins Research and Non-Research Evidence Appraisal Tools	Rapid Critical Appraisal Checklists (Melnyk & Gallagher-Ford, 2015)	AXIS (Downes, Brennan, Williams, & Dean, 2016)
		X	X		
	X	X	X	X	
			X		
		X	X	X	
		X	X	X	
		X	X	X	
			X		
		X	X	X	
		X	X		
				X	
				X	
	X		X	X	
		X			X

if this is a study on the most appropriate radiation therapy for breast cancer patients and all the authors are nurses, you may want to question whether they should have consulted a radiation oncologist to ensure that they are not missing any recommended treatments. You may also want to consider the author's stake in the results of the paper. For example, if the research is testing a new technology and one of the authors is the inventor of the technology, this may bias the results. They should state clearly somewhere their conflict of interest, but even if they did, you may want to interpret the results with caution.

Take a look at the abstract. This provides a very general description of the study, the reasons for conducting it, and the results. Abstracts are helpful to get a sense of the article overall and can be a good reference to look back at if you are reviewing many studies and need to quickly refresh your memory. A structured abstract is presented in the same way as a scientific paper. These can vary but usually include a background/introduction section, purpose/objective, methods (how the study was done), results (what the researchers found), and discussion/conclusion (where the authors interpret the meaning of the results in the context of existing literature). It is important to bear in mind that while the abstract is very helpful, it does not provide enough information in and of itself to determine the quality of the results. Therefore, you need to continue your critique of the strengths and weakness of the study and the way it was conducted to determine its utility in a larger context. Before we begin, take a few minutes to read the article.

Step 3: Appraise the Article

We will use the Joanna Briggs Institute Critical Appraisal Tools for use in JBI Systematic Reviews Checklist for Analytical Cross Sectional Studies (Moola et al., 2020), which can be found at https://joannabriggs.org/sites/default/files/2019-05/JBI_Critical_Appraisal-Checklist_for_Analytical_Cross_Sectional_Studies2017_0.pdf.

1. Inclusion/Exclusion Criteria

The first question asks whether the inclusion/exclusion criteria were clearly defined. When you set up a study, you want to make sure that the inclusion criteria are clear; in the example of nurses Sarah and Margaret, Margaret failed to ensure that the participants weren't already doing some kind of meditation. It is easy to see how this may affect the results; if some participants were already doing meditation, it is conceivable that the intervention may have less of an effect. In the study we are critiquing in this example (Gonzalez-Mercado et al., 2018), the stated objective is "To examine the health related quality of life (HRQOL) experienced by 79 Puerto

Rican adults during cancer treatments." By looking at the objective of the study, you can get an idea of what kind of participants they should recruit. They should be Puerto Rican adults currently receiving cancer treatment(s). Looking at the methods section under "design and sampling," you find the specifics of the inclusion/exclusion criteria (see Figure 4.3).

Methods

Design and Sampling

This study used a descriptive, cross-sectional design. A convenience sample (N = 79) was drawn from Hispanic Puerto Rican men and women with any cancer diagnosis all undergoing cancer treatments as outpatients. The participants were included if they: had a diagnosis of cancer; had received at least two or more rounds of therapy; and, were at least 21 years of age or older. Data collection was conducted in June 2016. The recruitment and data collection of study participants took place at two ambulatory cancer treatment facilities located in San Juan, Puerto Rico.

Figure 4.3 | Sampling strategy reported in Gonzalez-Mercado et al. (2018).

The authors describe the inclusion criteria as being "diagnosis of cancer; had received at least two or more rounds of therapy; and were at least 21 years of age or older." They do not list exclusion criteria, but many times these are not needed if they are implicit in the inclusion criteria (i.e., if you said inclusion criteria includes that the participant must have a diagnosis of cancer, then you would not need to list exclusion criteria as being those without a diagnosis of cancer). However, the authors might want to have excluded those that had not had their last round of therapy recently or those with the diagnosis of cancer many years ago (i.e., in remission). These inclusion criteria are very broad and include any type of cancer at any stage. By limiting to those receiving outpatient treatments, the authors may have helped narrow the types of participants included in the study, even though it wasn't explicitly stated in the inclusion/exclusion criteria. For example, the range of severity of the cancer may be somewhat limited in outpatients, and if they recruited from a treatment center, this may have helped ensure that the patients were currently receiving care and that the cancer diagnosis was recent. Because the authors did not list these specifically, we are left to assume that this was the case; this helps underscore the importance of very specific, detailed inclusion criteria.

You may question why the study authors decided not to include adults 18 and older or why they decided to only sample Puerto Ricans living in Puerto Rico. In all research it is important to remember that whatever you decide to do for your study design, you should be able to clearly describe the rationale when you write up your manuscript.

2. Sample and Setting

The second question in the JBI checklist asks about the sample and setting. This is important because, ultimately, the reason you are reading the study is to determine how useful it is to you. In this case, if you were thinking about investigating the HRQOL of Puerto Rican cancer patients who live in the United States, this article might be a good starting point. This study would allow you to compare the experiences of Puerto Ricans who live in Puerto Rico versus those in the United States. However, if your study question was about the HRQOL of all Americans undergoing cancer treatment, you may feel that this study is too specific to apply the results to your study.

Another question you may want to ask is whether the sample size is appropriate for the study objectives. Earlier in the chapter we mentioned the importance of doing a sample size calculation. The reason that you need to do a sample size calculation is to determine if you have enough people in your sample to detect an effect from the intervention. Let us think back to the example with nurses Sarah and Margaret. If meditation caused a drop in BP of 40 points, that would be a very large effect, so perhaps you do not need very many people, and even with Margaret's small sample of five people, she might be able to detect the effect. However, more often than not, we do not expect a large effect and want to be able to test for even a small effect. In such cases, we would need many more people to detect a small effect. A sample size calculation uses statistical methods to help you determine whether you have enough people (if your samples are people) to detect whether your intervention made a difference. You may also hear this referred to as a *power analysis*. There are two types of errors that can occur; a power analysis reduces the chance of making these errors (see Table 4.3). The first is a type 1 error, which says that the intervention works when it did not (false-positive), and the second is a type II error, which says that the intervention did not work when really it did (false-negative). The power is the percent chance that you will be able to detect an effect that did not occur by chance. While people may use these terms interchangeably, a sample size calculation tells you how many people you need in your sample based on a given power and effect size, and a power analysis tells you what power you achieved given a certain sample size and effect size. It is generally accepted that you should try to achieve a power of .80 (or 80%).

Table 4.3 | Types of Errors

Error	Also Known As	Description
Type 1	False-positive	Coming to the conclusion that an intervention worked when it did not.

Table 4.3 | Types of Errors

Type II	False-negative	Coming to the conclusion that an intervention did *not* work when really it did.

If the authors do not calculate a sample size, you must consider how the sample size affects the validity of the results. The Central Limit Theorem tells us that a general rule of thumb would be that you need at least 30 people in each arm of a study, but this does not account for the complexity of the study (Israel, 1992). One way to think of this is that the simplest study will require at least 30 participants, and the sample size will increase as the complexity of the study increases (the more factors being considered, etc.).

In this case, the authors report that this is a pilot study. Many people believe that a pilot study does not require a sample size calculation because sometimes the point of a pilot study is to help with future sample size estimation (in a larger study). Guidelines for pilot studies do exist (Hertzog, 2008). Furthermore, you may think that in a cross-sectional study, you would not need a sample size calculation; you are describing a sample, so there is no effect to detect. However, you can see in the data analysis section that the authors do compare the men and women, so they do need to conduct a sample size calculation to determine whether they have sufficient numbers to detect differences between groups. In fact, some argue that you should always be very clear when conducting a pilot study about what your future goals are; that is, if you state you are conducting a pilot study, then you should include clear information about the planned larger studies in the future that will be informed by the pilot (Arain et al., 2010).

3. Reliability and Validity

Reliability and validity refer to the ability of the instrument to accurately measure the thing it is trying to measure (validity) and the ability to measure it consistently (reliability; Golafshani, 2003). The two main types of validity are internal (is the study reporting results that are valid?) and external (can they be applied to other groups?; Delgado-Rodríguez & Llorca, 2004). There are many ways to describe reliability and validity, including *selection bias* (are they recruiting people in a way that may influence the outcomes?) and *information bias* (trouble with the way the information is collected). Information bias is a broad category that includes *recall bias* (when the participant can't quite

Validity:
The ability of an instrument to accurately measure the thing it is purported to measure.

Reliability:
The ability of an instrument to measure the same thing consistently.

remember) and problems with measurement (does the instrument used accurately measure what they think they are measuring?) (Delgado-Rodríguez & Llorca, 2004; Golafshani, 2003).

For now, let us think about the survey as presented in this study. Suppose you were interested in the effects of medication therapy on hypertension. If you were to conduct a survey and you asked all of your colleagues, "What do you think about therapy for hypertension?", you may get a wide variety of results—some people may think you are talking about psychotherapy, others massage therapy, others physical therapy. You would have poor validity because you did not ask the question in a way where you would be sure to get people's thoughts about medication therapy. You would have poor reliability because, depending on whatever recipients happened to be thinking about when you asked them, they may answer you differently each time. This is why it is important to make sure that whenever a survey instrument is used, it has been tested for reliability and validity; there are tests that can be done by researchers to verify the reliability and validity of an instrument. In this study there is a section of the methods called "Quality of Life – FACT-G" where the authors discuss reliability and validity of the Spanish version of the instrument they used to measure HRQOL in the study.

The authors report on the instrument's psychometric properties and report r's of −0.54 for Mood State, −0.47 for Performance Status (Cella et al., 1998). Guidelines suggest that a strong correlation would be a correlation coefficient of $> .30$ (Hemphill, 2003), so for each of these you see that the validity is good, indicating that the instrument is actually measuring Quality of Life, as they suggest. They also report 0.18 to show a lack of a relationship with the social desirability subscale, which they report was expected (although it was not explained). *Cronbach's alpha* is a measure of reliability that is generally considered acceptable if it is between .75 and .90 (Gliem & Gliem, 2003). This test reports an overall Cronbach's alpha that is within this accepted range, demonstrating reliability of this instrument. Another option is to look up the reference given for the paper that tested the reliability and validity to gain additional information and verify what is reported here.

Thus, this study is based on an instrument that has had some sound testing for reliability and validity. Not much information is given on how patients were recruited, so you do not know about selection bias. (For example, if the person recruiting tended to ask patients who looked sad if they would like to participate, then the HRQOL scores could be negatively skewed or vice versa for upbeat patients.) An inherent bias of surveys is that data is self-reported, so you do not know whether people tended to report things as being better or worse than they actually were. (This is why studies that collect objective data are preferred.) These limitations are mentioned in the discussion, which gives some assurance that the authors have considered these things as they interpreted the results of the study.

4. Measurement of the Condition

This question is asking how you know that you recruited for the correct population. You see that the information on diagnoses and treatment were self-reported (see Figure 4.4), so you do not have objective assurance that the patients actually had the reported condition. However, as we have previously discussed, this fear can be allayed by the fact that the participants were recruited at an outpatient oncology treatment center. In the example with nurse Margaret, you really have no way of knowing whether Margaret recruited appropriately because the diagnosis was self-reported and not confirmed appropriately. In Sarah's study, you have more assurance that she has appropriately recruited because she confirmed the diagnoses following appropriate clinical guidelines.

Quality of Life - FACT-G

The Functional Assessment of Cancer Therapy- General (FACT-G) QOL questionnaire instrument was developed by Cella and colleagues specifically for cancer survivors (12). The FACT-G version 4 includes 27 statements containing 4 subscales: physical (e.g. "I have lack of energy; 7 items), functional (e.g., "I sleep well"; 7 items"), social/family (e.g., "My family have accepted my illness"; 7 items) and emotional well-being (e.g., "I feel sad"; 6 items) were rated by the patients who were asked to indicate the degree to which they felt that each statement was true during the preceding week. Each item is anchored by a five-point Likert-type scale response ($0 =$ not at all, $1 =$ a little bit, $2 =$ somewhat, $3 =$ quite a bit, or $4 =$ very much). Scores on the FACT-G can range between zero and 108. After appropriately reverse coding items, scoring for this scale was computed by adding the individual item scores, and dividing by the number of items answered. Higher scores represent better HRQOL (13).

The FACT-G has been validated with Spanish-speaking cancer patients, with good psychometric properties including: significant negative relationships with a related concept of Mood state (Brief Profile of Mood States; $r = -0.54$) and Performance Status (Eastern Cooperative Oncology Group Performance Status Rating; $r = -0.47$); and an anticipated lack of relationship with social desirability (short form of the Marlowe-Crowne Social Desirability Scale; $r = 0.18$). The overall Cronbach's alpha was 0.89 (14).

Demographic Data and Health Form—Demographics included the respondent's age, gender, ethnicity, and years of education. Information on diagnosis and treatment modality was also obtained. The research assistant obtained that information from the participants' self-report on the demographic form.

Figure 4.4 | Reliability and validity of instruments in the article by Gonzalez-Mercado et al. (2018).

It should be noted that a survey is always inherently flawed because the data collected are subjective. However, this does not mean that surveys are not useful; it just means that you want to keep that subjectivity in mind when considering how much weight to put on the study. If you have another study that is a randomized controlled trial of good quality that gives different results, you might put more weight on it than the results of the survey.

5. Confounding Identified, and 6. Confounding Addressed

A *confounder* is something that potentially skews the results. Questions 5 and 6 ask if the confounding factors were identified and whether they were addressed. There is the potential that the confounders were addressed without being identified or that they were not identified and not addressed, so you should answer both of these questions even if the answer to number 5 was no.

Identifying confounders can be difficult because you have to think about whether there was something outside the situation that might have influenced the results. In the example with nurses Margaret and Sarah, circadian rhythm is a potential confounder because it causes a person's BP to fluctuate throughout the day; this could mean that the authors may have potentially included some people as being hypertensive who actually were not, or they may get a decreased BP if they measured later in the day (with or without the intervention) and come to an erroneous conclusion. Ideally, the study authors would have thought about this and addressed the confounders in some way—for example, by changing the study design or through statistical analyses that account for confounding factors. Because many confounders can be addressed through statistical analyses (e.g., multivariate regression), it would have helped if the study authors had collected more specific information about where the patient was in the cancer process. A woman on her first treatment of chemotherapy may have had a very different HRQOL than someone who had had several rounds of chemotherapy already and was battling a relapse. Although this was not accounted for and the authors do not specifically refer to it as a confounder, the authors do allude to this being a problem.

A confounder is often something that we as the readers would be unlikely to know. For example, if the data were collected at a very low-quality facility and participants were aware their treatment was suboptimal, they may report that they have very low HRQOL, but this is something that you would not know unless the authors mentioned it. The authors of this study did not list that they identified or accounted for any confounders. A potential confounder might have been that the survey was administered at the treatment center. Because participants were actively receiving (or about to, or just finishing) treatment, this could potentially cause them to be thinking about their cancer, or feeling very sick or anxious and having a more negative outlook on their HRQOL than they would if they were at home or in another setting, causing the results to be skewed.

7. Outcome Measures

The appropriate measurement of outcome measures needs to be evaluated. In the study about hypertension, you would ask how Margaret and Sarah measured BP. Did they follow the appropriate guidelines for measuring BP? Did they use a calibrated cuff? Was the patient relaxed and not talking prior to and during the measurement? Was the arm elevated? All of these are important in ensuring accurate measurement. Whereas question 4 asked us to consider how the diagnosis was measured (in this example, appropriate diagnostic guidelines), this question is talking about the outcome (a reduction in BP). In the study by Gonzales, you see that the diagnosis was self-reported, and the outcome was measured using Functional Assessment of Cancer Therapy-General QOL questionnaire (FACT-G).

You have considered the reliability and validity of the tool. You must also consider whether the tool is appropriate for measuring what the authors are intending to measure. It is helpful to go back to the beginning and remind yourself of the objective of the study; in this case it was "To examine the health related quality of life (HRQOL) experienced by 79 Puerto Rican adults during cancer treatments." If this is the objective, then the selected tool should be able to measure the health-related quality of life. If you now return to the methods section to read the description of the instrument, it says, "The Functional Assessment of Cancer Therapy-General (FACT-G) QOL questionnaire instrument was developed specifically for cancer survivors." So, while the objective of the study was to study patients with active cancer treatment, the instrument was developed for "cancer *survivors*." The question is, will the tool still be reliable and valid when it is being used in a related but very different population? This is something you have to decide for yourself. It is likely that if the objective was to measure something very similar (in this case HRQOL), then it is probably fine. However, if this was something that you were planning to do a study on yourself, and you really needed to know the answer, you might decide that you need to go back to the original publication on the instrument and figure out how closely the populations are related and whether you think this tool was used appropriately.

This may sound like a lot of work, especially if you are critiquing a large number of papers, but sometimes you have to do a personal mini-cost/benefit analysis. If this topic is something really important to you and your career or patients' lives are riding on the outcome, then you will not mind spending some extra time looking into it or recruiting some colleagues to help with your review. If this is just for your personal information about the quality of life experienced by Puerto Ricans undergoing cancer therapy, you may decide to trust the study authors that this is the best available tool to measure HRQOL in this population. Or, if you are writing a book chapter and you are not a cancer or HRQOL expert, and you picked this study to critique because a very kind colleague offered to allow you to do so, you probably are not going to need to spend any more time looking into the instrument.

Another important thing to consider at this point is the way the measurement was collected. Again, you need to look carefully at the methods. How was the survey administered? This should be in the section labeled "Data Collection." Studies should always mention human subjects' approval, often called the *Institutional Review Board* (IRB). An IRB helps ensure that studies are done in an ethical way. Researchers must receive approval to do research on humans or animals, and they should mention this somewhere in the paper, even if it is to say that the study was exempted from the IRB. Even in the instance of a survey, IRB approval is needed. For example, in this study if the authors had approached patients in a way that made the participants think that they would not receive treatment unless they completed the survey, they might have completed the survey and filled it out in the way they thought would allow the researchers to grant access to treatment. The IRB helps ensure that the study is carried out in a way where problems such as these do not arise.

When you think about how the instrument was administered, it is important to think about the way it was carried out. Did the researcher lead them to a private, quiet room and give them plenty of time to fill out the survey? Did they fill out the survey while receiving their chemotherapy? While they were waiting to be seen? Was it a combination of these things? It is important that the survey be administered consistently each time to help ensure that the results will be similar in each case. For example, if some people were given the survey during chemotherapy, they may be very uncomfortable and give a very negative view of their HRQOL. Their results may differ significantly from someone who is there for their first chemotherapy visit; by not administering the survey the same way each time, the potential for bias increases. In this instance, you do not know exactly what the study authors did because it is not described in detail. This would be something to consider as you think about the results of the survey.

8. Statistical Analyses

This question asks whether appropriate statistical analyses were used. This can be difficult for clinical nurses to evaluate. Fortunately, there are many helpful guides available on the internet. One of these by Jaykaran (2010) has a free flow diagram that helps you follow what to do from the study objective to the right statistical test (see Figure 4.5).

In the Gonzalez-Mercado study, the authors aim to describe the HRQOL scores of the participants. Starting at the top of the diagram, you see the first box on the left is "description of one group." Select this box and follow the line down. Looking at the Gonzalez-Mercado paper again, in the methods section, you read, "After appropriately reverse coding items, scoring for this scale was computed by adding the individual item scores, and dividing by the number of items answered. Higher scores represent better HRQOL." A number divided by another number is a *ratio*, so going back to the diagram, you pick the first box (R, I) for ratio and interval data. If you continue to follow the line down, it asks whether the data were normally distributed. Looking again at the Gonzalez-Mercado paper under methods, you see that the authors report that the data were not normally distributed. So according to the diagram, they should have reported a median and an interquartile range. Under the results section of "HRQOL" there is no interquartile range reported. Looking at Table 4.2 in the Gonzalez-Mercado paper, note that there is no interquartile range. So, you are left to decide—did the authors conduct the appropriate statistical test? In this instance, perhaps not technically. However, most of us reading this would probably not say the mean was inappropriate and in fact could be more clinically meaningful than a range.

Next let us look at the comparison of the HRQOL scores between men and women. If you follow the flow diagram starting at the top, this is a comparison of two groups (male versus female) ➜ unpaired groups (meaning the groups are not matched to represent each other in an intervention versus control study) ➜ ratio data interval data (the score of the FACT-G) ➜ non normal distribution (per the study authors) ➜ Mann-Whitney test. In the article by Gonzalez-Mercado, the authors report using the Mann-Whitney test, so you can feel assured that they have done the appropriate test in this instance.

Step 4:
Summarize the Results and Make a Decision

Now that you have finished appraising the article, you need to think about your overall assessment of the article. First, just think about whether, based on the quality of the evidence presented, this article is a good one to include, whether it should be excluded, or whether you need to do a little more digging to decide what to do (like in the instance we discussed where you may want to look up some references cited in the article to confirm what the authors report). On the JBI instrument,

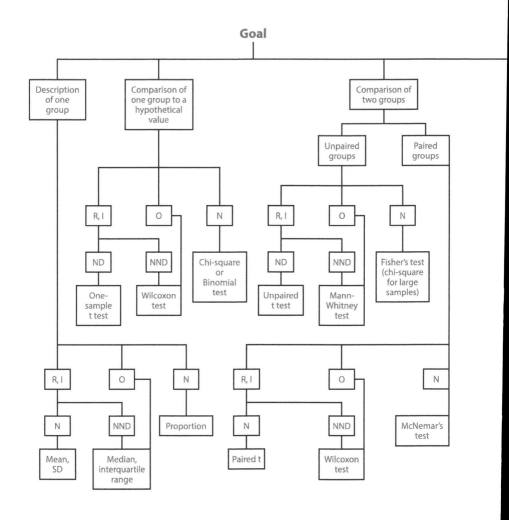

R, I = Ratio and Interval data | O = Ordinal data | N = Nominal data
N = Normal distribution | NND = Non normal distribution

Figure 4.5 | How to select the appropriate statistical test from Jaykaran (2010).

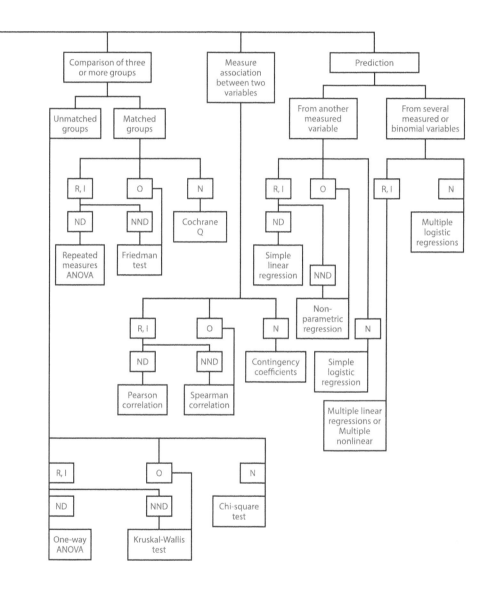

there is a checklist to the right of each question so that you can answer "yes," "no," "unclear," or "not applicable." As you have seen, the answer to this is somewhat subjective, so it may also be helpful to make some notes so that you can decide how important the "yes," "no," or "unclear" really is (see Table 4.4).

Table 4.4 | Summary of Results of Critique

Criteria From JBI Tool	Criteria Satisfied?	Notes	
		Strengths	Weaknesses
1. Inclusion/ exclusion criteria	Yes	Likely to select for intended population	Not very precise
2. Sample and setting	Unclear	Sample size > 30	Did not do a sample size calculation
3. Reliability and validity	Yes	Used a well-tested instrument	The tests for reliability and validity were also on a small sample size
4. Measurement of the condition	Unclear	Recruited from a location likely to select for the right population	Self-reported diagnoses
5. **6.** Confounding	No	None reported	Recruiting from a cancer treatment center may have negatively skewed the results
7. Outcome measures	Yes	Used a validated tool for measuring HRQOL in cancer survivors	The population being treated were current cancer patients (as opposed to survivors) Methods are not well described regarding the administration of the survey
8. Statistical methods	Yes	Appropriately used Mann-Whitney test	Authors could have presented interquartile ranges for scores if data were not normally distributed

In this study, and in likely every study, you will find that there are some flaws that you are willing to live with. The primary goal is to see what the strength of the evidence is, so even if the evidence is not strong you still may want to use it if it is the best available evidence. In the instances where there are many studies of the same type on a topic, you may want to throw out the lower-quality studies. If you find a study that is critically flawed, you should definitely not use it because the results are meaningless. In the example about Margaret's study, that would be the kind of study you would not use because there are just too many flaws to really accept the results as meaningful. Overall, the Gonzales study has some flaws, but the results are likely to be valid for this population despite these issues.

The next question to ask is whether the sample is similar enough to the population in your own PICO question for the results to be able to be generalized to your population. For example, if you had the same PICO question as Margaret and Sarah but you wanted to only look at inpatient adults, you would need to consider whether these studies would be similar to your population. In the case of a study with an intervention, you need to ask yourself whether the intervention is something that you can replicate. In this case, could you replicate the meditation class that Sarah provided and be able to collect data for such a long time span? This is very unlikely to be the case. (Even for outpatient studies it is unrealistic.) In research, we refer to this as the *feasibility* of the study. It is important to think about the scope of your project and how likely you are to be able to finish it or sustain the project. If you are considering replicating the study, you should think about the study's feasibility.

Finally, you should think about the costs and benefits of the study. Continuing with our example of Sarah's study, if the meditation were free and likely to reduce BP even a little bit, then it could be worth trying to replicate it. However, if you had to pay someone to organize the class, incentivize participants, hire a research assistant to check and record the BP, and a statistician to analyze the results, then you would probably want the payoff to be more than just a modest reduction in BP. This is one reason that many studies are surveys; they are low-cost and you can gather a lot of data. Each of these points should be considered and will ultimately help you decide whether to include the study in your final synthesis of the literature.

Drawing a Conclusion

After you have finished appraising the quality of all the studies you are looking at for your topic that you think may help you answer your PICO question, it is time to synthesize the results and make a decision about what to do next (see Figure 4.6). If you can reasonably conclude that the results of your literature review have answered your question, you can implement a change in practice (hence the term *evidence-based practice*). If you are unable to answer your PICO question, you can consider conducting a research question to answer your question. (This is assuming you have done a good literature search that returned the appropriate results.) If your initial PICO question was in response to a problem in your practice (e.g., a unit has high nursing turnover, and the purpose is to understand how to reduce it, or a hospital has a high rate of nosocomial infections and is looking for ways to reduce them), then you implement this change in practice as a quality or practice improvement activity.

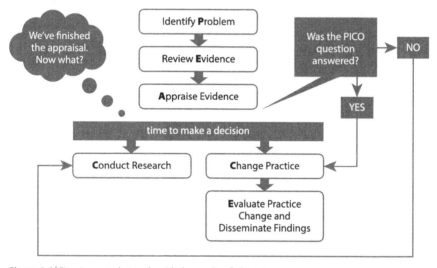

Figure 4.6 | Figuring out what to do with the results of a literature review.

Summary

Conducting an appraisal of the literature is like any other skill; it takes time to develop and requires practice. However, it is important that nurses become competent at critically appraising evidence to ensure that they base their practice on the best available evidence. It is no longer acceptable to practice something because that was what we were trained to do; evidence changes, and we must stay abreast of the most recent practices and research (McMenamin et al., 2019). Furthermore, by spending the time upfront to critique an article, you can be confident that your project is sound as you move forward.

When you first begin appraising articles, you may feel like you are spending an inordinate amount of time on these first three steps (developing a strong PICO question, conducting the evidence review, and appraising the evidence). However, rest assured that you will save yourself a lot of time in the long run because you will avoid the mistakes that others have made and build on the best available evidence.

Rather than replicating interventions that have been done with very little effect or sustainability, you will conduct research or change practice in a way that is rigorous, feasible, and sustainable.

Review Questions

1. Why is it important to consider the quality of each related study prior to conducting a research study or a quality improvement activity?

   Answer: Not all studies are of the same quality, which may lead to incorrect conclusions about a particular outcome. By appraising the evidence, you can be assured that you are not conducting a research study or changing practice based on incorrect information.

2. How does one find an appropriate appraisal tool?

   Answer: First, read the article to determine the type of study being appraised. Next, search for a tool that matches the type of study. The Joanna Briggs Institute and the Critical Appraisal Skills Programme are good places to start, but there are many others (refer to Table 4.2).

3. How does one determine whether the methods of a study are appropriate and the conclusions justified?

   Answer: By following the selected checklist, you can make an informed decision about whether the evidence is solid. Be sure to consider contextual factors, such as whether the authors have the needed expertise to interpret the results of the study or have competing interests, as well as the importance of the decision you will make based on the results.

4. What does one do with the results of a study, and does it matter if the study is flawed?

   Answer: Almost all studies are flawed, but it is important to consider how critical the flaws are. Some minor lapses in the way the study is reported are probably OK to overlook, but a critical design flaw would render the results meaningless. Summarizing the results will allow you to decide whether there is sufficient evidence to make a practice change or whether further research is needed.

5. Why are the first three steps of the PEACE model so important when they take up so much time?

   Answer: They take time, but without them your own work may be severely flawed. The first three steps are foundational in ensuring that your own research study or practice change is evidence-based, not redundant, and sustainable.

References

Arain, M., Campbell, M. J., Cooper, C. L., & Lancaster, G. A. (2010). What is a pilot or feasibility study? A review of current practice and editorial policy. *BMC Medical Research Methodology.* https://doi.org/10.1186/1471-2288-10-67

Brouwers, M. C., Kho, M. E., Browman, G. P., Burgers, J. S., Cluzeau, F., Feder, G., Fervers, B., Graham, I. D., Grimshaw, J., Hanna, S. E., Littlejohns, P., Makarski, J., Zitzelsberger, L., & AGREE Next Steps Consortium. (2010). AGREE II: Advancing guideline development, reporting and evaluation in health care. *Journal of Clinical Epidemiology, 63*(12), 1308–1311. https://doi.org/10.1016/j.jclinepi.2010.07.001

Buccheri, R. K., & Sharifi, C. (2017). Critical appraisal tools and reporting guidelines for evidence-based practice. *Worldviews on Evidence-Based Nursing, 14*(6), 463–472. https://doi.org/10.1111/wvn.12258

CASP. (2017). CASP Checklists. *Critical Appraisal Skills Programme.* Available at: https://casp-uk.net/casp-tools-checklists/

Cella, D., Hernandez, L., Bonomi, A. E., Corona, M., Vaquero, M., & Shiomoto, G. (1998). Spanish language translation and initial validation of the functional assessment of cancer therapy quality-of-life instrument. *Medical Care, 36*(9), 1407–1418.

Charan, J., & Biswas, T. (2013). How to calculate sample size for different study designs in medical research? *Indian Journal of Psychological Medicine, 35*(2), 121–126.

Delgado-Rodríguez, M., & Llorca, J. (2004). Bias. *Journal of Epidemiology and Community Health.* https://doi.org/10.1136/jech.2003.008466

Dijkers, M. (2013). Introducing GRADE: A systematic approach to rating evidence in systematic reviews and to guideline development. *E-Newsletter: Center on Knowledge Translation for Disability and Rehabilitation Research.* Available at: http://www.mitaeroa.com/pdf/c101.pdf

Downes, M. J., Brennan, M. L., Williams, H. C., & Dean, R. S. (2016). Development of a critical appraisal tool to assess the quality of cross-sectional studies (AXIS). *BMJ Open.* https://doi.org/10.1136/bmjopen-2016-011458

Fineout-Overholt, E., Melnyk, B. M., Stillwell, S. B., & Williamson, K. M. (2010). Evidence-based practice, step by step: Critical appraisal of the evidence part III. *American Journal of Nursing, 110*(11), 43–51. https://doi.org/10.1097/01.NAJ.0000390523.99066.b5

Gliem, J. A., & Gliem, R. R. (2003). Calculating, interpreting, and reporting Cronbach's alpha reliability coefficient for Likert-type scales. *2003 Midwest Research to Practice Conference in Adult, Continuing, and Community Education.*

Golafshani, N. (2003). Understanding reliability and validity in qualitative research. *The Qualitative Report. 8*(4), 597–607.

Gonzalez-Mercado, V. J., McMillan, S., Pedro, E., Tirado-Gomez, M., & Saligan, L. N. (2018). The health related quality of life of Puerto Ricans during cancer treatments: A pilot study. *Puerto Rico Health Sciences Journal, 37*(1), 46–51.

Hemphill, J. F. (2003). Interpreting the magnitudes of correlation coefficients. *American Psychologist, 58*(1), 78–79. https://doi.org/10.1037/0003-066X.58.1.78

Hertzog, M. A. (2008). Considerations in determining sample size for pilot studies. *Research in Nursing and Health, 31*(2), 180–191. https://doi.org/10.1002/nur.20247

Higgins, J. P. T., Savović, J., Page, M. J., Elbers, R. G., Sterne, J. A. C. Chapter 8: Assessing risk of bias in a randomized trial. In Higgins, J. P. T., Thomas, J., Chandler, J., Cumpston, M., Li, T., Page, M. J., Welch, V. A. (editors). Cochrane Handbook for Systematic Reviews of Interventions version 6.0 (updated July 2019). Cochrane, 2019. Available from www.training.cochrane.org/handbook

Israel, G. D. (1992). *Determining sample size.* University of Florida IFAS Extension. https://www.tarleton.edu/academicassessment/documents/Samplesize.pdf

Jaykaran, C. (2010). How to select appropriate statistical test? *Journal of Pharmaceutical Negative Results, 1*(2), 61–63. https://doi.org/10.4103/0976-9234.75708

Joanna Briggs Institute. (2019). *Critical appraisal tools.* http://www.cebm.net/critical-appraisal/

Lee, M. C., Johnson, K. L., Newhouse, R. P., & Warren, J. I. (2013). Evidence-based practice process quality assessment: EPQA guidelines. *Worldviews on Evidence-Based Nursing, 10*(3), 140–149. https://doi.org/10.1111/j.1741-6787.2012.00264.x

McMenamin, A., Sun, C., Prufeta, P., & Raso, R. (2019). The evolution of evidence-based practice. *Nursing Management* (September), 14–19. doi:10.1097/01.NUMA.0000579000.09987.b0

Melnyk, B. M., & Gallagher-Ford, L. (2015). Implementing the new essential evidence-based practice competencies in real-world clinical and academic settings: Moving from evidence to action in improving healthcare quality and patient outcomes. *Worldviews on Evidence-Based Nursing, 12*(2), 67–69. https://doi.org/10.1111/wvn.12089

Moola, S., Munn, Z., Tufanaru, C., Aromataris, E., Sears, K., Sfetcu, R., Currie, M., Qureshi, R., Mattis, P., Lisy, K., & Mu, P-F. (2020). Chapter 7: Systematic reviews of etiology and risk (Appendix 7.5: "Checklist for analytical cross-sectional studies"). In Aromataris, E., Munn, Z. (Editors). *JBI Manual for Evidence Synthesis.* Retrieved from https://synthesismanual.jbi.global

Wang, J. G., Kario, K., Park, J. B., & Chen, C. H. (2017). Morning blood pressure monitoring in the management of hypertension. *Journal of Hypertension, 35*(8), 1554–1563. https://doi.org/10.1097/HJH.0000000000001379

Whelton, P. K., Carey, R. M., Aronow, W. S., Casey, D. E., Collins, K. J., Dennison Himmelfarb, C., DePalma, S. M., Gidding, S., Jamerson, K. A., Jones, D. W., MacLaughlin, E. J., Muntner, P., Ovbiagele, B., Smith Jr., S. C., Spencer, C. C., Stafford, R. S., Taler, S. J., Thomas, R. J., Williams Sr., K. A., Williamson, J. D., & Wright, J. T. (2018). 2017 guideline for the prevention, detection, evaluation, and management of high blood pressure in adults: Executive summary: A report of the American College of Cardiology/American Heart Association Task Force on Clinical Practice Guidelines. *Hypertension, 71*(6), 1269–1324. https://doi.org/10.1161/HYP.0000000000000066

Zodpey, S. P. (2004). Sample size and power analysis in medical research. *Indian Journal of Dermatology, Venereology and Leprology, 70*(2), 123–128.

PEACE MODEL

P | **PROBLEM IDENTIFICATION**

Formulate the clinical question (**PICO**):

- **P** | Patient Population
- **I** | Intervention
- **C** | Comparison of Intervention
- **O** | Outcome

E | **EVIDENCE REVIEW**

Review evidence relevant to your clinical question by searching databases.

A | **APPRAISE EVIDENCE**

Appraise the evidence that appears highest in the hierarchy of scientific evidence for its quality and applicability to practice.

C | **CHANGE PRACTICE OR CONDUCT RESEARCH**

If evidence is sufficient, embark on improvement project to address practice change.

If evidence is insufficient to warrant practice change, conduct research.

E | **EVALUATE AND DISSEMINATE FINDINGS**

Evaluate the impact of the implemented practice change and research results.

Disseminate findings through publication, oral, and poster presentations.

5

CHANGE PRACTICE

–Alexandra N. Shelley, MS, RN-BC, FNP-BC
Jessica O'Brien Gufarotti, MS, RN, AGCNS-BC, PCCN
Haofei Wang, DNP, RN, NEA-BC

KEYWORDS | PHRASES
EBP mentor, elevator speech, evidence-based practice, implementation, pilot phase, policy, practice change, stakeholders, sustain planned change

CHAPTER OBJECTIVES
After studying this chapter, learners will be able to:

1. Identify steps to engage key stakeholders in practice changes.
2. Describe steps of implementation plans for practice changes.
3. Identify strategies to sustain practice changes.

Introduction

Finding and critically appraising scientific research can be a challenge, but once you have completed these steps, you may face even more challenges—namely, translating the evidence you have found into practice. If you have determined, based on your review and critical appraisal of evidence, that there is a difference between the state of current practice in your clinical setting and what is published as evidence as the best practice, you have found an *evidence-practice gap* (National Institute of Clinical Studies, 2003). You may decide that you need to revise the current practice or introduce a completely new practice to address this gap and ensure that the practice is evidence-based to enhance healthcare quality, improve patient outcomes, and reduce costs (Melnyk & Fineout-Overholt, 2019). In this chapter, we review and demystify the major steps in planning and implementing evidence-based practice (EBP) change, and we provide strategies that can facilitate the process and set you up for success.

Key Terms

Active stakeholder: Someone who has a key role in making a project happen (Fineout-Overholt et al., 2011).

EBP Change Team: The team responsible for planning and implementing an EBP change.

EBP mentor: Someone with expertise in EBP who provides knowledge and support (Melnyk & Fineout-Overholt, 2019).

Elevator speech: A clear, brief, and persuasive message that can spark another's interest in your project.

Evidence-practice gap: Lapse between the publication of evidence and its implementation into practice (National Institute of Clinical Studies, 2003).

Implementation: Putting something into effect (Edie, 2018).

Organizational policies: Guidelines, procedures, and principles that are intended to underpin the work and decisions made by an organization's employees so that the organization's goals can be achieved (Melnyk & Fineout-Overholt, 2019).

Passive stakeholder: Someone who may not be actively involved in the project but who could promote or stymie its success (Fineout-Overholt et al., 2011).

Pilot phase: Small-scale implementation to prove the feasibility, scalability, and safety of a proposed project.

Key Steps to Implementing Practice Change

Setting out to change practice is no easy task, even when armed with robust, high-quality evidence. Following a systematic process can help ensure success and sustainment of practice changes. Major steps for changing practice include identifying and engaging key stakeholders and then forming an EBP Change Team, acquiring approvals for practice change, formulating a comprehensive implementation plan, holding a launch meeting and carrying out the implementation plan, and finally, sustaining the change (Gallagher-Ford et al., 2011).

Identify and Engage Key Stakeholders and Members of EBP Change Team

Essential to the success of implementing changes are project stakeholders. *Stakeholders* have long been defined as "any group or individual who can affect or is affected by the achievement of the organization objectives" (Freeman, 1984, p. 46). For the sake of nursing practice change, *active stakeholders* are those who are directly affected by or directly affect the new practice. Making a list of stakeholders should be the first step in planning for a change. Active stakeholders in nursing practice changes often include, unsurprisingly, nurses. However, in healthcare, nursing practice changes are not always confined to affecting practicing nurses. In fact, it is rare that nursing practice changes do not affect others, so give some thought to who else may have an active "stake" in the change. Think of other departments and disciplines that could be affected by a change in practice. For instance, if you want to implement a new evidence-based early mobilization program, you will want to include representatives from the physical therapy department in planning and implementing the changes. An early mobilization program that includes physical therapy consultation would affect the workflow of physical therapists, and the contributions of physical therapists in formulating the design and implementation of the program could affect its success. You will want to include these active stakeholders (or a representative from the department) as team members of your *EBP Change Team*, the team responsible for implementing the practice change. When stakeholders are involved in developing the plan for implementation, they are more likely to support the change.

Not all stakeholders have equal stake. In the context of implementing new practices or revising current practices, there are also *passive stakeholders*—those who may not be directly affected by the change but can help the change succeed or hinder its success (Fineout-Overholt et al., 2011). Think of who might fit this definition. A common example might be nursing leadership. Leadership can influence the success of a practice change because supporting the change as a priority promotes overall buy-in from other hospital team members (Li et al., 2018). A director of nursing may not be actively involved in the implementation of an early mobilization program on a unit, but the director can promote its success through communicating that it is a priority and setting expectations for nurses on the unit that it is a necessary practice change to improve patient care outcomes. Another example of passive stakeholders are those responsible for the oversight of nursing practice and policy within your organization. This may include a director of nursing practice or a nurse practice committee that helps provide insight into the feasibility, applicability, and design of practice changes and can assist in disseminating changes and guidelines or policies to help sustain the

EBP. While these passive stakeholders need to buy into the change and should be kept informed of the progress during implementation, they may not necessarily need to participate as active members on your EBP Change Team.

Having a dedicated EBP Change Team that is inclusive of both clinical experts and *EBP mentors* is key to a successful implementation of any EBP project. Clinical experts and EBP mentors have advanced knowledge and skills in EBP and implementation strategies and often have a foundational background in organizational and individual change (Melnyk & Fineout-Overholt, 2019). Clinical experts and EBP mentors have past experiences and can share lessons learned, and they can help shape the visions for the future state of evidence-based projects within organizations. They will act as your sounding board and coach to driving change. Some examples of clinical experts and EBP mentors include:

- Nurse researchers
- Advanced practice nurses (nurse practitioners, clinical nurse specialists)
- Nursing professional development specialists
- Healthcare quality improvement specialists
- Nurses with previous EBP implementation experience
- Nurse leaders (clinical or administrative)

Identify one or more of these clinical experts or mentors to include on your EBP Change Team, and communicate with them frequently about any uncertainties or barriers that you face throughout your practice change project.

Engaging Stakeholders and Team Members

Building a case for change will help gain buy-in from your stakeholders. Articulating your vision for the practice change and the supportive rationale is essential in convincing others that the change is worth the time and resources needed to implement it (Melnyk & Fineout-Overholt, 2019). This can also help generate enthusiasm and a sense of urgency around the change. Having a pitch or elevator speech prepared when you are first engaging your team members and stakeholders is helpful, so that key messages can be delivered succinctly and convincingly. Table 5.1 includes important points to cover during your *elevator speech*, along with some helpful tips in getting your point across (Agency for Clinical Innovation, 2015).

Table 5.1 | Crafting Your Elevator Speech

Key Points to Cover	Helpful Tips
What is the current state?	What is currently the routine practice that exists in your clinical area where you have identified an evidence-practice gap? Explain what that current practice is, and perhaps include why or how you identified it as a problem.
What is the desired state?	Remember to look beyond the immediate state post change. Think about what you want the future, sustained state to look like. Include a vision for improved outcomes.
What is the practice change?	What practices (behavior, actions, workflow, environment design, etc.) will need to change, and what does the new practice look like?
Why is the practice changing?	Provide a brief summation of your evidence review and appraisal. Again, you may emphasize here the urgency to improve outcomes.
What are the potential benefits of change?	Remember to leverage all potential points of beneficial impact. These include benefits to patients/families, employees, and your organization.
Who will the changes affect?	Think active and passive stakeholders, but also think about who the proposed change will have a secondary impact on (i.e., supply chain, the bed management/admitting team, providers.).
What are the measures of success?	Using data can be one of the most compelling resources to captivate your stakeholders' attention. When putting together your elevator speech, have an idea of data measures ready to show that you have thought about determining the short- and long-term impact of the change.

To leverage buy-in for practice change, it is important to consider your methods for creating excitement about your vision. This will help promote motivation and engagement of potential team members who not only believe in your cause but also will be eager to promote and execute the change. Consider using a catchy phrase that captures your practice change. For an early mobilization program, you might use the phrase "Let's Get Moving!" and perhaps start off your pitch with an inter-est-generating headline, such as, "How would you like to decrease the length of stay of our ICU patients?" Other methods of engaging stakeholders include taking the time to listen and understand their concerns and interests and seeking their input into establishing specific steps of the implementation plan, such as outcome measurement (Fineout-Overholt et al., 2011).

As you are engaging your stakeholders and recruiting your EBP Change Team members, it is important to consider and address potential barriers that could hinder future engagement with your project and vision. Stakeholder resistance or second thoughts could result from a number of factors, including reluctance to change traditional practice; unfamiliarity with EBP values, outcomes, or principles; and misconceptions about the time and effort it takes to implement change (Melnyk et al., 2011). Involve your EBP mentors when considering these barriers. They will be able to help you identify the potential hurdles and facilitators that will improve retention of stakeholders and team members. Anticipating resistance to change or reluctance for involvement from the start will allow you to prepare appropriately to effectively manage disinclination.

Gain Approvals for Implementation

Administrative approval: Gaining administrative and leadership support for your project vision is an important step to consider during the beginning stages of implementing an evidence-based project. Successful implementation of EBP is heavily influenced by leadership, as formal leaders can help sustain new processes and are essential for overall hospital staff buy-in (Li et al., 2018). A good rule of thumb is, after you have identified those who will be involved in the project as EBP Change Team members and you have developed an organized, shared vision of the practice change, seek administrative support and approval (Melnyk & Fineout-Overholt, 2019). In doing this, you are ensuring the practice change aligns with organizational goals and visions and setting up your project for support, success, and sustainability. Examples of administrators to obtain approval from would be unit or departmental managers, directors, and, depending on your project scope, the chief nursing officer. This approval process can be intimidating and challenging to navigate, and your knowledge of what approvals are needed from an organizational level may be limited, so discuss with your immediate supervisor what is required at your organization.

Approval of professional governance councils and committes: As stated earlier, many organizations have governance structures or committees that provide oversight to nursing practice. While these structures may be helpful to have during your change implementation for extra support and guidance, they also will likely need to approve nursing practice changes prior to implementation. Ask to be added to a meeting agenda of any committees that must provide approval, or speak directly with the committee leadership to determine the process for approving practice changes in your organization.

Develop an Implementation Plan

Implementation simply means putting something into effect. Spend some time on formulating and writing a detailed project management plan that lays out your process for implementing the change. Dedicating time to plan and prepare will clarify the aim, steps, timeline, and roles for your project team. Table 5.2 lists and describes the specific components to include in your implementation plan (Agency for Clinical Innovation, 2015).

Table 5.2 | Crafting an Implementation Plan

Project Plan Component	Component Description
Specify project objectives/goals	This will ensure that all members of your EBP Change Team are working toward the same goals and help clarify the objectives so that there is a shared understanding about how your team will know if the project has been successful. Consider using the "SMART" acronym in writing out project goals (**S**pecific, **M**easurable, **A**ttainable, **R**elevant, **T**imely).
Formalize EBP Change Team member roles	Clarify roles and responsibilities of each team member so that the implementation stays on track. Examples of formalized roles can include a sponsor, project lead, clinical lead, education lead, and project champions. Make sure you are specific about what each role entails.
Develop project timeline	The project timeline is going to be one of your most valuable resources for keeping you on track. Your timeline may vary from project to project depending on the size, scope, and structure of the change you're implementing. Some of the most important components of a project timeline are tasks, deliverables, deadlines, and most importantly, the expected time it will take for each task (Bunner, 2016). Include in your timeline a formal kickoff date and a plan for ongoing periodic check-ins with your stakeholders and EBP Change Team members to monitor implementation progress.

continues

Table 5.2 | Crafting an Implementation Plan *(cont.)*

Project Plan Component	Component Description
Determine measurements	Determining how you will evaluate your project aims should be done before implementation. Having baseline data to compare to post-implementation data enables measurement of implementation success. You can also include measurements that you will collect during implementation for ongoing monitoring to discuss with your Change Team during check-ins.
	Measures may be process-driven or outcome-driven. For example, in an early mobilization program, you may measure how often the process of moving patients out of bed is completed (process measure), as well as the length of stay or ventilator days of patients who participated in the program (outcome measures). Include in your plan whether you will need to create a process to collect this data or whether you can tap into data that is already collected, for example, from your quality department.
Specify and describe steps of implementation	Lay out the action steps you plan to take to actually operationalize the new practice, and consider including some of the following (Cullen & Adams, 2012):
	• Education/communication of the change. Multimodal is best (e.g., live, virtual), and include different shifts/times to accommodate
	• Validation of new practice competence through skills redemonstration, knowledge exam, and more
	• Rollout of new materials or equipment to match new practice*
	• Printed resources, manuals, quick-reference guides, flowcharts, or algorithms*
	• Periodic reminders or practice prompts
	• Feedback to stakeholders about change progress
	• Recruit and train change agents, such as champions, to help propel the change forward
	• Incentives and recognition for observed practice change by stakeholders

*Pilot the change first

Tips for Seamless Planning

- Depending on your organization, you may find it valuable to ask your local leadership team if there is any project management software the organization utilizes and explore whether this may aid in your project implementation.

- If you find yourself stuck or unsure of how to create a project plan or timeline that can be accessed in a way that is valuable and seamless, think about the technology most of us use everyday, such as a smartphone or computer. Create shared calendars or live documents where you can see changes made by other members in real time.

- Before you decide on your measurements, do some research into the metrics that are already being collected at your organization and see if you can access the data. For example, most healthcare organizations routinely measure and report patient satisfaction data, such as from the Hospital Consumer Assessment of Healthcare Providers and Systems survey, and quality and patient safety data, such as patient falls and central line–associated blood stream infections.

- More often than not, your timeline or plan may require multiple revisions during your project as priorities shift, barriers are identified, and competing priorities arise.

Other Planning Considerations

There are other important considerations to address when planning for EBP change, including change resistance, workflow and work environment specifications, and alignment with organizational policy.

Resistance to Change

Think about a time where a practice change has occurred on your unit. Were you openly ready to accept and adopt the proposed change? Or did you give some pushback? Did you need to be sold on how the change would affect your nursing practice and workflow as well as your unit and patient outcomes? Consider these past experiences of resistance as you plan implementation, and anticipate possible facilitators to help combat change resistance. Thinking of this and incorporating facilitators into your implementation plan ahead of time will serve you well during the implementation stages. Table 5.3 describes why some people may resist the change you are trying to implement.

Table 5.3 | Reasons People Resist Change

Reasons for Resistance	Facilitators to Reduce Resistance
Misunderstanding why change needs to occur	If stakeholders do not clearly understand why the change is important, resistance will occur. This is particularly important to consider when discussing change with nurses who have mastered their practice with decades of nursing under their belt.
Fear of the unknown	This is one of the most common reasons to resist change. People will generally only move toward the unknown if you give them great reason to believe that moving forward will have positive outcomes.
Lack of knowledge, expertise, or skill	Change challenges us. It's an inevitable part of inviting something new for people to question their ability to succeed. Providing positive feedback and reassurance will help people trust their abilities to move forward.
Attached to an old practice/process	Many people who are connected to a process or practice they have mastered are hesitant to learn a new way of doing things. Consider providing sound rationale, data, and outcomes to sell why the new way is better than the old. From there, if you are still meeting resistance, you can break down why the old way is no longer the gold standard.
Difficulty trusting the change process	We have all experienced a time when an idea or new process has not succeeded. Remind people that this is OK! With all new things come trials and tribulations that we can only grow from. Growing pains are an inevitable part of growth and improvements.
Believing the proposed change is only a trend or a fad	Explore the evidence with these staff members. Show them data, outcomes, and metrics. The important thing about EBP is that someone else has already demonstrated that the practice can be successful.
Not being consulted first	People like knowing about changes that could *potentially* affect them, before the change becomes a reality. Informing people of best practices before they are implemented could help increase buy-in.
Lack of communication	There is no such thing as too much communication. People like to stay in the know and be informed, especially when the change affects them and their job directly.
Disruptions to routine	Exploring or functioning outside of comfort zones can be one of the biggest barriers to accepting change. Helping people see the potential for success when they step outside their box will increase acceptance.

Table 5.3 | Reasons People Resist Change

Burnout	Our personal lives, careers, and mental capacity all have a ceiling for the amount of change that can be processed during a certain time period. Understanding that burnout and exhaustion are real will help you connect not only with those affected by the change but also your teammates and stakeholders.
Perceptions of the status quo	Perception versus reality. People who feel the change will hold no benefits for them will be resistant to offer their support. Similarly, if people feel the change only benefits one department or unit, they may in turn become resentful and have negative effects on your progress. Be sure to discuss the positive impact the change can have on all areas during implementation to prevent toxicity.
Cannot visualize benefits	People want to know how the outcomes of the change will benefit them, their unit, and their patients. Use this opportunity to share your vision, the evidence, and, if need be, give them your elevator speech. There is a reason people make a career out of selling products. They help people see into the future and grasp the *why* behind the *what*.

Adopted from Rick, 2011. Copyright 2019 by the American Psychological Association.

Workflow and Work Environment

You may find there is more resistance to practice change if the plan for implementation is not compatible with existing processes or the environment in which stakeholders practice. Think about how you can integrate the change in practice into the existing workflow. If a change or disruption in workflow is necessary, think about how you can facilitate understanding of the change through an algorithm or flowchart that can be easily referenced by stakeholders. For example, for an early mobilization program, you could try to incorporate the new process for consulting physical therapy to enroll early mobilization patients into an existing interdisciplinary rounds process to minimize the addition of a separate process. Then you could create a flowchart and checklist that would help to prompt nurses and physical therapists how to select patients who are eligible and the actions to take to enroll them in the program.

You should also think about possible disruptions in the work environment. A common example of this might be the need for new or alternative supplies or equipment. While some evidence-based changes may in and of themselves be changes in materials, it is often likely that practice changes require some new materials to be carried out. In an early mobilization program, there may be a need for additional or specialized patient mobility equipment. Think about what your material needs might be during the planning stages so you can match your vision for practice change with the need for new supplies or equipment.

Organizational Policy Alignment

Before formally implementing a practice change, it is best to review relevant policies in your organization to determine whether any gaps exist between the planned practice change and the way in which the policies are currently written. *Organizational policies* pertain to the guidelines, procedures, and principles that are intended to underpin the work and decisions made by an organization's employees so that the organization's goals can be achieved (Melnyk & Fineout-Overholt, 2019). In your organization, these may be digital documents, or hard copies may be made available for your access. Ensuring that your organization's policies allow for the EBP that you plan to implement can help sustain the new practice by providing information that guides nurses on how to carry out the practice and by demonstrating that the practice is supported by the organization. Make sure you contact and collaborate with the director of nursing practice/policy at your organization to determine whether policy change is needed and to obtain the director's assistance in carrying out a policy amendment or addition if a change is warranted. Keep in mind that some organizations require that a pilot phase (see the upcoming "Launch a Pilot" section) be implemented with measurement of outcomes to determine organizational value and applicability prior to policy changes.

Carry Out the Implementation Plan

To ensure a successful implementation, you need to, first, hold a launch meeting to engage all stakeholders and discuss project deliverables, tasks, responsible person(s), and timeline; and then, to launch a pilot to prove the viability of the project.

Hold a Launch Meeting

The launch meeting is the official kickoff that sets the tone for your project. This is the opportunity for you to get the EBP Change Team and stakeholders on the same page, build excitement, share and finalize your implementation plan, and begin operationalizing the change. Before your meeting, make sure you establish what your main priorities are to review and what your desired outcomes are from getting your team and stakeholders together. To keep your launch meeting productive, be sure to create a well-defined agenda, stay organized, and be prepared to guide the conversation. An ideal launch meeting will have the majority of stakeholders (active and passive) or stakeholder representatives and EBP Change Team members in attendance. Ensure that a project sponsor can attend, and consider including those from other departments who could be affected by the change in the future. During your meeting, be clear about the timeline and, before finalizing your steps for implementation, elicit additional input. Before you leave the meeting, ensure that teammates who are responsible for deliverables are aware of their responsibilities, and set deadlines for those deliverables. Also be sure that all who attend the meeting are aware of the implementation plan that will be carried out, a formal implementation date, and what the responsibilities of each team member are on that date. More tips for planning your launch meeting are included in the following sidebar.

Tips for Planning Meeting Success

- Reserve a dedicated space for the meeting. Staff lounges and nurses' stations can be noisy and distracting.
- Send your agenda in advance via an email reminder for the meeting at least one week before.
- Print copies of materials for meeting attendees; include items such as the agenda, implementation plan, and implementation timeline.
- Remember that you will most likely need to meet with your EBP Change Team at recurring intervals after the launch of your project, so it is recommended to preschedule follow-up meetings to give team members plenty of advanced notice.
- Ask a team member to take detailed minutes and share with meeting attendees afterward so that you have a complete record of any decisions made or follow-up needed.

Launch a Pilot

A *pilot phase* is a small-scale implementation to prove the feasibility, scalability, and safety of a proposed project. This could include testing the viability of a new idea or, in this case, an EBP that has proven to work and result in positive outcomes at outside organizations. Implementing change generally requires making alterations in workflows and providing clinician education, which takes time. During your pilot phase it is important to remember that success will be founded on clarity of objectives, communication, and expected or desired outcomes. It is normal for people to have some degree of uncertainty or reluctance to accept your proposed change (refer to Table 5.3), so remind your team and stakeholders that the pilot phase is merely to prove the practicality of your project and not necessarily to deliver all the anticipated outcomes. Encourage team members, active stakeholders, and passive stakeholders to ask questions and address concerns early on and throughout your pilot phase. This will give you and the EBP Change Team the opportunity to make any necessary revisions and alterations to your project plan that you may not have anticipated. Remember, don't be discouraged if you find that many changes need to be made to your original project plan. Most successful projects go through multiple revisions to adapt to actual workflows and practice. All in all, it is strongly suggested that you and the EBP Change Team consider incorporating a pilot phase into your project plan regardless of the scale of your project. Depending on the project and the intervention you are proposing, the EBP Change Team will need to determine the need for either a small-scale or a large-scale pilot phase to test the proposed change. The following sections illustrate the different approaches between a small-scale and large-scale pilot phase.

Small-scale pilot phase: The EBP Change Team is piloting a new EBP to reduce hemolyzation rates in the emergency department (ED). The proposed change is to attach IV connection tubing to the newly inserted IV prior to collecting blood samples versus the current practice of connecting a vacutainer directly to the hub of the newly inserted IV to collect blood samples. To pilot the change, you and the EBP Change Team work with the laboratory manager and three nurses during a one-week period. The three nurses will collect the blood samples using the new method and mark the blood tubes to alert the laboratory manager so he can assess the outcomes of proposed change. The remainder of the ED will continue practicing using the current method. After one week, the EBP Change Team, the three nurses, and the laboratory manager meet to assess the practicality of the proposed change.

Large-scale pilot phase: The EBP Change Team is piloting a new EBP to reduce falls in the organization. The proposed change is to hang in each patient's room fall risk signage that is tailored to individual needs. To pilot the change, the EBP Change Team tests the change on one medical-surgical unit during a one-month period. The EBP Change Team is testing two changes during this pilot phase, which includes a test of the fall risk signage in the nursing workflow and a test of which securement device works best to display the sign. The remainder of the organization will continue to practice using the current method of placing yellow fall risk bands on high-risk patients. After one month, the EBP Change Team, the unit nurse manager, and nurses from the pilot unit meet to discuss moments of success, opportunities for improvement, and feasibility of the proposed change.

Sustain Change

The key to sustaining changes in practice is following your plan and timeline for implementation. Follow up frequently with your EBP Change Team to ensure that the plan is being carried out appropriately and on time.

Monitoring Implementation Progress

One of the best ways to ensure that a practice change is sustained is through monitoring the progress of the implementation. Many times, this may be done through collecting process metrics to determine whether the process of the new practice is being followed by practitioners. This is often done through chart audits, direct observations, or self-report tools, such as surveys. Ongoing monitoring of implementation using these methods provides evidence of whether the change is being implemented and information about barriers that need to be addressed for the change to be sustained (Agency for Clinical Innovation, 2015).

Eliciting and Sharing Feedback

Collecting feedback from stakeholders and the EBP Change Team is essential to inform implementation progress and to determine whether amendments in the implementation plan are needed. Sometimes, this feedback comes in the form of resistance to the change; under many conditions, resistance need not be seen as a barrier to overcome but instead an opportunity to refine the plan for change (Erwin & Garman, 2010). Keep this in mind as you elicit feedback, as to not discourage the plan to implement EBP and progress toward the goal of improvement.

Sharing feedback from progress evaluation with the EBP Change Team and stakeholders is also important; this can motivate the stakeholders to continue the implementation plan or can provide information about how efforts to implement the change need to increase to meet desired targets (Agency for Clinical Innovation, 2015).

Celebrate Wins

Recognizing and celebrating success as the practice change is being implemented can be another powerful motivator for stakeholders to continue with the implementation plan. Celebrating positive trends in metrics, both process- and outcome-related, as well as recognizing individuals for their contributions in carrying out change implementation can be done in a variety of ways. Newsletters, email announcements, and "shout-outs" during huddles or meetings are simple and impactful ways of providing meaningful recognition.

Outcome Metrics

The ultimate goals of implementing EBP are to enhance healthcare quality, improve patient outcomes, and reduce costs (Melnyk & Fineout-Overholt, 2019). To know whether these goals are being achieved through the implementation of a new practice, outcomes must be measured and compared to baseline measurements of the same outcomes.

Expansion of Pilot Phase

If a pilot phase was a part of your implementation and you determined that the practice change is applicable and feasible, consider how you will expand to other clinical areas and units in the organization. Expansion of the practice throughout other areas, using the same planning and diligence as the pilot phase, will help with organizational uptake and sustainability of the new practice.

Policy Updates

Organizational policy updates can be useful interventions in supporting the integration of EBP changes (Cullen & Adams, 2012; Gallagher-Ford et al., 2011). As discussed earlier in this chapter, organizations may have different requirements as to what qualifies and how to constitute a policy change. Seek out the director of nursing practice/policy at your organization to determine actions needed to integrate practice changes into policy.

Summary

Changing practice to ensure evidence is translated at the bedside can be challenging, but with a well-thought-out plan and organized implementation, paired with tenacity and strategies to sustain the changes, one can be successful in leading EBP changes. Following systematic steps and continuous reevaluation of the process will ensure effective changes in practice in clinical settings.

Review Questions

1. You are implementing a new evidenced-based project on your unit to help monitor patients for the development of hospital-acquired delirium. You include your unit's team of physician assistants (PAs) because this change will directly affect their practice. For this project, the PAs would be:

   A. Active stakeholders

   B. Passive stakeholders

   C. EBP mentors

   D. Clinical experts

   Answer: A. Active stakeholders. The unit's team of PAs would be active stakeholders because they will be directly affected by and directly affect the new practice. Often, nursing practice changes affect multiple disciplines outside of nursing, so it is important to think of all team members who would have an active stake in the change.

2. Building a case for practice changes is important to gain buy-in from stakeholders. Sharing your vision and convincing others the practice change is worth their time will help generate enthusiasm around the change. Having a(n) _____ prepared will help you share your vision in a way that's concise yet convincing.

   A. Catch phrase

   B. Notification email/memo

   C. Elevator speech

   D. Presentation

   Answer: C. Elevator speech. Having an elevator speech prepared when you are first engaging with your team members and stakeholders will be very helpful when trying to recruit and excite your team. Your elevator speech should cover topics like, What is the current state? What is the desired state? What is the practice change? Why is the practice changing? What are the potential benefits of the change? Who will the change affect? What are the measures of success?

3. When developing a detailed project plan for how you and the team will implement a proposed change, it is important to ensure that all members of the EBP Change Team are working toward the same goals. Writing out project goals using the SMART format will help keep objectives clear and concise. SMART stands for:

   A. Strict, Measurable, Attainable, Related, Together

   B. Specific, Manageable, Actionable, Related, Timely

   C. Strict, Measurable, Achievable, Relatable, Together

   D. Specific, Measurable, Attainable, Relevant, Timely

   Answer: D. Specific, Measurable, Attainable, Relevant, Timely.

4. Testing a proposed evidenced-based project on a smaller scale ensures feasibility, scalability, and safety of the proposed plan. This small-scale implementation is called the:

   A. Technical working plan

   B. Trial run

   C. Pilot phase

   D. Test launch

   Answer: C. Pilot phase. A pilot phase is a small-scale implementation to prove the feasibility, scalability, and safety of a proposed project. Implementing change generally requires making alterations in workflows and providing clinician education. It also allows time for clarifying objectives, communication, and desired outcomes.

5. Monitoring implementation progress is one of the best ways to ensure practice change is sustained. Assessing sustainability can be done through:

   A. Chart audits

   B. Collecting process metrics

   C. Direct observation

   D. All the above

   Answer: D. All the above. Collecting process metrics, completing chart audits, and directly observing the area(s) affected by the practice change are great methods to ensure the change is being sustained throughout implementation. Ongoing monitoring will provide evidence of whether the change is effectively being implemented and information about barriers that need to be addressed for the change to be sustained.

References

Agency for Clinical Innovation. (2015). *Implementation guide: Putting a model into practice.* https://www.aci.health.nsw.gov.au/__data/assets/pdf_file/0007/291742/Clinical_Innovation_Program_Implementation_Guide.pdf

Bunner, A. (2016). *Project timelines: Why they're so important.* https://www.clarizen.com/project-timelines-why-theyre-so-important/

Cullen, L. L., & Adams, S. (2012). Planning for implementation of evidence-based practice. *Journal of Nursing Administration, 42*(4), 222–230.

Edie, A. H. (2018). Organizing an evidence-based practice implementation plan. In T. Christenbery (Ed.), *Evidence-based practice in nursing: Foundations, skills, and roles* (pp. 197–213). Springer Publishing Company, LLC.

Erwin, D. G., & Garman, A. N. (2010). Resistance to organizational change: Linking research and practice. *Leadership & Organization Development Journal, 31*(1), 39–56.

Fineout-Overholt, E. M., Williamson, K. M., Gallagher-Ford, L. B., Melnyk, B., & Stillwell, S. (2011). Evidence-based practice, step by step: Following the evidence: Planning for sustainable change. *AJN, 111*(1), 54–60.

Freeman, R. E. (1984). *Strategic management: A stakeholder approach.* Pitman.

Gallagher-Ford, L. M., Fineout-Overholt, E. B., Melnyk, B., & Stillwell, S. (2011). Evidence-based practice, step by step: Implementing an evidence-based practice change. *AJN, 111*(3), 54–60.

Li, S., Jeffs, L., Barwick, M., & Steven, B. (2018). Organizational contextual features that influence the implementation of evidence-based practices across healthcare settings: A systematic integrative review. *Systematic Reviews, 7,* 72.

Melnyk, B., & Fineout-Overholt, E. (2019). *Evidence-based practice in nursing & healthcare: A guide to best practice.* Lippincott Williams & Wilkins.

Melnyk, B. M., Fineout-Overholt, E. B., Gallagher-Ford, L., & Stillwell, S. (2011). Evidence-based practice, step by step: Sustaining evidence-based practice through organizational policies and an innovative model. *AJN, 111*(9), 57–60.

National Institute of Clinical Studies. (2003). *Evidence-practice gaps report. Vol. 1.* https://www.worldcat.org/title/evidence-practice-gaps-report-volume-1/oclc/57004951

Rick, T. (2011). *Top 12 reasons people resist change.* https://www.torbenrick.eu/blog/change-management/12-reasons-why-people-resist-change/

PEACE MODEL

P | **PROBLEM IDENTIFICATION**

Formulate the clinical question (**PICO**):
- **P** | Patient Population
- **I** | Intervention
- **C** | Comparison of Intervention
- **O** | Outcome

E | **EVIDENCE REVIEW**

Review evidence relevant to your clinical question by searching databases.

A | **APPRAISE EVIDENCE**

Appraise the evidence that appears highest in the hierarchy of scientific evidence for its quality and applicability to practice.

C | **CHANGE PRACTICE OR CONDUCT RESEARCH**

If evidence is sufficient, embark on improvement project to address practice change.

If evidence is insufficient to warrant practice change, conduct research.

E | **EVALUATE AND DISSEMINATE FINDINGS**

Evaluate the impact of the implemented practice change and research results.

Disseminate findings through publication, oral, and poster presentations.

6

CONDUCT RESEARCH

–Allison A. Norful, PhD, RN, ANP-BC | Kevin D. Masick, PhD

KEYWORDS | PHRASES
research design, quantitative analysis, hypothesis, sampling,
scales of measurement, data analysis

CHAPTER OBJECTIVES

After studying this chapter, learners will be able to:

1. Describe components of C (**C**onduct research of the PEACE model).
2. Describe the purpose for doing research.
3. Identify the steps to conduct research.
4. Design a research study utilizing the PEACE model.

Introduction

At this point you have determined there is a gap in the literature that warrants a research study. The next logical step is to determine how you will conduct your research. There is no one right way to conduct research. Every decision you make must be carefully thought out, as certain methodological decisions affect future actions. Whether you are conducting research for the first time or are an experienced researcher, there is always an opportunity to learn something new. Conducting research can be overwhelming and confusing. The purpose of this chapter is to provide an overview of how to get started by focusing on common questions and specific examples that drive the research process. This chapter aims to walk you through the process of developing your research plan, including its design, sample, and analysis, as well as how to obtain all required approvals to ensure you conduct an ethical study. Of note, this overview only begins to tap into some of the initial decisions you will need to make in the planning of your study. We recommend that you reach out to a research mentor in your institution who can guide decisions that are specific to your study design and analysis.

Institutional Review Board (IRB)

I Want to Conduct a Research Study. Do I Need Approval From an Institutional Review Board (IRB)?

There are a few required hurdles that must be passed prior to stepping out in the world of conducting research. Every researcher with an end goal of completing a study and possibly publishing must submit for review by an institutional review board (IRB). Now you may be thinking that you are conducting quality improvement research as a means to get around this requirement. This would be incorrect, as any institutional research must be presented to the IRB. The main purpose of the IRB is to ensure that your research abides by the ethical and legal standards for conducting research. Most IRBs require some form of training to ensure you understand how to properly protect human subjects and maintain protocol with the Health Insurance Portability and Accountability Act. Easily accessible online modules meet most IRB requirements. Inquire with your organization to determine exactly what training is needed prior to IRB protocol submission and the initiation of any study. For more information and to access online training programs, visit the Collaborative Institution Training Initiative (www.citiprogram.org).

From an IRB perspective, there are generally three different types of research studies: full board, expedited, and exempt. A *full board review* example would likely be a clinical trial or a study that poses a significant risk to patients. For any research study that is complex or requires multiple variables to evaluate, the board would want to ensure that participants are protected and there are no legal/ethical issues within the study. An *expedited review* is traditionally a less complex study that can often be approved by one or two individuals. These types of studies post minimal risk to participants. For example, an anonymous nursing survey poses minimal risk to participants. These types of research studies often contribute to new knowledge or expand on previously existing knowledge to the scientific community where data may already exist, or there will be interactions with participants to collect future data. An *exempt study* is a research study done within the confines of your organization for the purpose of quality improvement/performance improvement where the data that are being analyzed often already exist, and there will be no interaction with participants to collect new data. This may include the analysis of de-identified electronic health record data or a QI project where the data are aggregated at the unit or hospital level.

What Do I Have to Submit to the IRB to Gain Approval?

Every IRB has organization-specific documents that need to be completed. Currently, most of this documentation is electronic and can be accessed online. Take a few moments to familiarize yourself with the questions that the IRB is asking you.

Next, each study you submit for IRB approval needs a document called a protocol, which describes the purpose of the study, methodology, means of recruiting participants, data collection plan, and plans to analyze the data. Following is a step-wise approach to fulfilling each of these protocol sections.

Designing a Research Study

Why Am I Conducting Research? What Is the Purpose of Research?

The primary goal of research is to create new knowledge. Therefore, as mentioned in previous chapters, it is imperative to conduct an extensive literature search to review current evidence and understand what is already known about the process, practice, or phenomenon that you intend to study. Many nurses become overwhelmed with the idea of starting from scratch to invent something new. However, keep in mind that you are building upon what is already known. Most studies that have been previously conducted will list further research implications and what is yet to be discovered. Familiarize yourself with current publications including the study purpose, targeted population, methodology, and primary results. Publications also may list limitations of their studies, which will provide hints as to what may have gone wrong during the investigation or any potential bias that the results include. By grasping the successes or shortcomings of previous studies, you will be able to avoid such pitfalls in your own study.

It is also important to take the time to reflect on why you want to conduct a study and how much if any impact your results would have. Research moves science forward whether results demonstrate statistical significance or not. We learn from past studies as to what works and what doesn't work, which is important to keep pursuing further inquiry. Conducting research does warrant a considerable amount of time, effort, and resources, so be sure that your potential study findings are worthwhile for the population you will study, your key stakeholders, and your own research team.

Leadership Support and Team Resources

Your management team and peers are important stakeholders that can really support your desire to conduct research. Gaining buy-in will help to speed up the process of approvals when seeking data or access to an intended sample. Transparency is key when explaining your study, its intentions, and the risks and benefits of your results and findings. Prepare an elevator speech that identifies the gap in the literature and how you intend to build new evidence.

How Do I Write a Research Question/Hypothesis?

The PICO question you have already developed will be the ideal starting point to fine-tune your research question. At this point you already have a general idea of who (population) and what (area of inquiry). The next question to ask yourself is why. Stemming from your literature review or your own clinical practice and observation, you likely already suspect the answer to your own research question. In other words, you hypothesize that x will lead to y. A *hypothesis* is an explanation for an observation, phenomenon, or scientific problem that can be tested by further investigation. The hypothesis includes a prediction about independent and dependent variables. An *independent variable* (IV) is the cause or something that is actively or passively changed or compared. Examples include clinical practice processes, educational interventions, and different healthcare disciplines or settings. The *dependent* variable (DV) is the effect or the impact that the independent variable has on particular outcomes and can be measured (e.g., blood pressure, mortality rates, patient satisfaction scores). Keep in mind that not every research study involves independent and dependent variables. There are times when you're conducting research where you may not be able to manipulate or change a variable, so you end up exploring relationships between multiple DVs.

There are different types of hypotheses and research questions. Some hypotheses look to examine causal inferences between variables, and others explore relationships. The type of hypothesis/research question you write will dictate the statistical analysis of your results. Whether you are exploring causal inferences or relationships, the framing of the question is similar. First, a *simple hypothesis* is a prediction of a causal inference between an independent and a dependent variable. Example: Smoking cigarettes (IV) causes lung cancer (DV). *Complex hypotheses* examine the causal inferences between two or more independent variables or two or more dependent variables. Example: Morbid obesity (IV) increases risk of mortality (DV) and decreased self-reported quality of life (DV). A *null hypothesis* predicts that there is no causal inference between the two variables. Example: A researcher may believe that a commercial-based diet will not lead to significant weight loss. An *empirical hypothesis* tests differences between groups, often involving different independent variables. Example: Surgical patient education about wound care before surgery reduces infection rates significantly greater than education performed at hospital discharge. When formulating your hypothesis, it is important to clearly define your variables and be specific and concise. If you take on variables that are two vague or broad, your results may not be applicable to

HINT!

Do not pose your hypothesis as a question but rather concisely state your prediction about the relationship or causal inference between variables.

similar groups or deemed invalid. Example: Holistic modalities post-surgery yield better patient outcomes (too vague). This is better: Orthopedic surgical patients who undergo aromatherapy after surgery will have a shorter length of stay.

Is My Hypothesis Testable?

As you begin to define your variables and draft your hypothesis, the type of study design you need to conduct will become increasingly clear. It *is* possible that there is not enough evidence to make a clear prediction just yet due to a lack of data that define your variables or help you make a prediction. You may need to conduct a preliminary study that aims to simply describe a phenomenon first and then support your intention to test a hypothesis. Let's walk through an example:

> *You are interested in reducing readmission rates of community dwelling older adults who are primarily cared for by family caregivers. Your literature search revealed that there is limited evidence about what resources family members need to feel adequately prepared to care for their loved one at home.*

In this case you want to obtain more knowledge to describe the experience of informal caregivers in the community. You also want to describe what types of resources the same family caregivers report are needed to care for their loved one. Collecting qualitative (e.g., perspectives, interviews, quotes about experiences) or quantitative (surveys, frequencies or percentages, empirical clinical information) data allows you to pursue your aims. A *qualitative descriptive study* is often conducted using in-person interviews or focus groups to illuminate previously unknown circumstances about an experience, setting, relationship, or phenomenon. Qualitative perspectives can help define your variables or identify different interventions to test or compare in a future study. A *quantitative descriptive study* involves the collection of empirical data to describe a population or phenomenon. For example, you may want to survey family caregivers about their ratings of the most important to least important resources that help them care for their loved ones. This could help you refine your potential independent variable. You could also collect hospital-level readmission rates describing the percentage of patients with family caregivers compared to those with formal caregivers. This may support readmission rates as your future dependent variable.

In some cases, both types of data are needed to create refined variables or future research questions. In this

HINT!

Descriptive studies are a great place to start for those who have conducted little to no research in the past. New researchers will have the opportunity to learn different methodologies to collect, manage, and analyze data while working on a research team.

case, a *mixed methods study* would be used to collect both quantitative and qualitative data. As an example, let's assume you decide to pursue a quantitative study
of informal family caregivers. After conducting a survey you determined that 85%
of family caregivers report that timely communication with a patient's primary
care provider is perceived as a critical resource. While this finding helps you focus
on a potential intervention, it also prompts additional questions. What mode of
communication? How often? What type of information needs to be communicated?
At this point you determine you need more information to decide what exactly your
intervention is most worthwhile to test. You decide to conduct in-person interviews
to obtain rich qualitative data and answer further questions needed to refine a
hypothesis.

I Have My Research Hypothesis.
How Do I Know What Research Design to Use?

As we have mentioned, there is no one way to conduct research. Some designs may
be more effective than others, but no design is superior to another. With all the
threats to the validity of your research, it still is possible to design a high-quality
study to answer your question. Research in general falls into one of three buckets:
preresearch, experimental, and quasi-experimental. Within those buckets, there are
many types of design choices you can make to reduce the threat to validity. These
could involve pre/post tests, between/within subjects design, or control groups. The
purpose of this section is to provide you with a decision tree to aid in the decision-making process for choosing the most appropriate research design for your
study. Prior to this decision tree, we outline some highlights of the three buckets of
research design and summarize the design features.

Preresearch is often used to begin to establish an issue to further research and
explore using more rigorous methods. This category of research is generally referred
to as *correlational research*. With correlational research, the main goal is to establish
that relationships exist but not dictate a cause-and-effect relationship. For example, you could conduct a correlational study to determine if there is a relationship
between nurse burnout by shift and nurses' intention to leave the organization. A
potential research question/hypothesis for this would be: Is there a relationship
between burnout and intention to leave? Within correlational designs, there are no
independent variables. You are not actively manipulating or changing a variable to
examine an effect. You are simply measuring variables to determine the extent to
which they are related. If you opt to design a more rigorous study and determine
a causal relationship through manipulating variables, then you would want to
explore experimental or quasi-experimental research. *Experimental research* is often
referred to as a laboratory study or the gold standard for conducting cause-and-effect
research. An example of a study using an experimental design would be an oncology

study evaluating the effectiveness of multiple medications on reducing tumors in patients. A key defining feature for an experimental design is that you must randomly assign participants to conditions. If you cannot randomly assign participants, then it is impossible to conduct an experimental design. As an alternative to experimental design, a *quasi-experimental* design is similar in nature to an experimental design. The only difference is that a quasi-experimental design does not require random assignment. An example of a quasi-experimental design could be to determine the impact that the scent of lavender has on patients. The only control you may have would be to select different units in a hospital. It would not be feasible to randomly assign patients to lavender versus no lavender, especially if patients share a room and one is exposed to lavender and the other is not.

In addition to the types of research design, there are other features to a research study you could implement to reduce threats to validity. Three such design features are pre/post tests, between/within subjects design, and control groups. The addition of pre/post tests allows you to collect multiple data points over the course of the study. In the initial design phase of your research you have the option to expose every participant to each part of the study or only expose participants to one condition. Lastly, you could add a control group to allow you to compare the results of your study to a group that does not receive the independent variable. You also have the ability to include some or all of the design features to enhance your study.

Research Methodology

At this point you have decided on a research design, and it is time to map out your methodology. Careful attention to your research methodology will help ensure that you avoid key pitfalls, increase the validity and reliability of your findings, and eliminate bias.

Population/Sample

You will first need to focus on your targeted population. When investigating a research question, it is nearly impossible to truly capture an entire population. Therefore, you investigate a sample or a *subset* that is representative of the population. Researchers often define specific inclusion and exclusion criteria that define who will be investigated. Is there a gender, race, age, or diagnosis that is specific to your research question? For example, the inpatient experience of an older adult may vary greatly from a pediatric patient. Will this influence your results or present a risk of bias?

Types of Sampling

Sampling participants falls into one of two buckets: a *probability sample* and a *nonprobability sample*. To determine which technique you need, you must know whether you have access to the entire population. If you do not know whether you have access to the entire population of interest, then it is not possible to do a probability sample. The purpose of the probability sample is to ensure that everyone has an equally random chance of being selected to participate in your study. A nonprobability technique means that not everyone has an equal chance of being selected to participate. There are many different types of sampling techniques you can use when selecting your sample (see Table 6.1). Picardi and Masick (2013) provide an overview of the various probability and nonprobability sampling techniques that are available to choose from.

The main requirement for selecting a sample using a probability sampling technique is that you must know or have access to the entire population of interest. Any probability sampling technique requires that the probability of including someone in your study is equal and that no one individual has a higher chance of being selected. Keep in mind that it is highly possible that you may not know or even have access to the entire population of interest, and that is perfectly acceptable. Nonprobability sampling techniques are quite common and used when the entire population is not known. The most common nonprobability technique is a *convenience sample*, which means that you collect data from participants based on whether you have access to this population. For example, if you are conducting research on sepsis patients, then the entire population would be any individual who has sepsis. The problem is that if you work at one hospital, then you don't know how to access sepsis patients at other hospitals, so you couldn't begin to do a probability sampling technique. This is where the location of interest becomes critical. Where are you conducting your research? A population is defined based on your criteria. If you are working in a community hospital and you want to do research on sepsis patients in your hospital, then your population of interest changes from sepsis patients around the world to sepsis patients within your hospital. This allows you to enhance your research design because you may know and have access to the entire sepsis population in the hospital. There are no advantages or disadvantages to deciding to use a probability versus a nonprobability sampling technique. The ultimate decision may be determined by accessibility to data or cost and time to obtain this information. See Table 6.1 for more on sampling techniques.

Table 6.1 | Sampling Techniques

Probability Techniques	
Simple random sampling	Basic sampling technique where random number is generated to select participants
Stratified random sampling	Sample is divided into subgroups and then participants are randomly selected
Cluster sampling	Sample is divided into geographic clusters, then randomly selected
Nonprobability Techniques	
Convenience sampling	Most common, where you collect data from participants you have access to
Snowball sampling	Sample based on using referrals to collect data from participants
Quota sampling	Sample selected based on a specific number of participants in a given group
Purposive sampling	Researcher specifically determines the participants that are typical of a given population

How Big of a Sample Do I Need?

The answer to this question involves multiple processes but can be solved utilizing a power analysis. The purpose of a *power analysis* is to determine how many participants you need in your study to find a statistically significant effect. The general acceptable level of power is 0.8.

This brings up other methodological issues to address, starting with how power is calculated. The formula for power is 1 – beta (type II error). Alpha is known as the type I error. Remember when we said that no research is perfect, and every decision you make could affect future actions? A *type I error* is when you say that you found a significant result when it does not exist, and a *type II error* is when you say no significant effect is found when one actually exists. This means that if you have a power of 0.8, your beta (type II error) is 1 – 0.8, or 0.2. In other words, a 0.2 beta means that 20% of the time, you will make a type II error, or 20% of the time you will say that you do not have a significant effect when you really do. You cannot directly control or set your beta level, but you can influence it based on the sample size. This is why it's important to conduct a power analysis and use the guideline of a power equal to 0.8 to find statistical significance. However, you can control your alpha level. Traditionally, to find significance, alpha is set at 0.05, 0.01, or 0.001. This means that your chance of making a type I error or finding a statistically significant effect when one does not exist is a 5%, 1%, or 0.1% chance, respectively. The moral of this story is to collect at minimum the necessary sample required using a power analysis. Once the ideal number of participants is determined, the next phase is to identify how you will recruit them.

Sample Recruitment

Your study will require a strategy for recruiting your sample of interest. This phase presents unique challenges that often can be tackled with proper planning based on the study's needs.

How Often Should I Have Access to My Targeted Sample?

You will need to ensure that your recruitment is feasible given your allotted time-line and resources. For example, recruiting patients with a rare condition may take longer because of the lack of hospital admissions of such patients over time. This will extend your timeline greatly and can be costly. On the other hand, if you are investigating a common chronic condition and work on a unit that is specific to this population, your recruitment may be easier because of the increased chance that you are consistently exposed to a patient who meets your criteria.

When and How Will I Recruit a Sample?

Recruitment can be performed in a variety of ways including in person, by tele-phone, by mail, or via email. The method often depends on whom you are recruit-ing and when the best time is to approach someone. For example, if you want to investigate the perspectives of nurses who work in the emergency department, you might consider getting permission to email all nursing staff explaining the study or hang a flyer in the staff breakroom. If you are investigating clinical outcomes of a surgical patient, it is important to explore ethical considerations. Is it best to recruit during presurgical testing as opposed to after a patient has already undergone surgery? There is no right or wrong answer to these questions, but your approach should be specific to what you intend to research.

Who Will Be Responsible to Recruit My Sample?

One researcher can only be present for so many hours in a day. Building a team that can carefully apply your criteria and flag potential participants in your study will greatly help to identify your sample in a timely fashion. Alternating days and shifts between your team members can increase the exposure of a potential sample. Map out a feasible schedule with your team to meet the goals of the study timeline.

Data Collection

What Type of Data Should I Collect?

In general, there are four different types of data that can be collected, and these are often referred to as *scales of measurement*, a hierarchy list where each scale above can have the properties of the scales below. The first two scales are considered qualitative scales and do not have quantitative properties. This means that you cannot calculate a mean or standard deviation for these two scales. The lowest scale of measurement is a nominal scale. The purpose of the *nominal scale* is to arbitrarily assign a number to a word or phrase to create a categorical or dichotomous variable. For example, gender and race/ethnicity are nominal scales where you could assign a value of 1 for females and 2 for males. You may be wondering why you would convert female or male to a 1 and 2 and not just leave it as female or male or F and M. Statistical software programs have the tendency to treat numbers more efficiently than words or phrases. Additionally, using numbers reduces the chances of different data entry. For gender, values of Female, female, and F would be treated as three separate variables. The next scale of measurement is an *ordinal scale*. It has no quantitative properties and was created for the purposes of providing a rank order. An example of an ordinal scale would be assigning a value for patients as they enter the emergency department. The first person who walks in would be assigned a 1, the second would be a 2, and so on. This numbering has no quantitative value because you do not know the time difference between the first and second patient.

The next two scales are quantitative scales where you can calculate means and standard deviations. The first quantitative scale is an *interval scale*. Its purpose is to provide an equal distance between each rating except for having a true 0. The most common interval scale is a *Likert-type rating scale* where there is typically a range of values between 1 to 5 or 1 to 7 or any other range. If you are measuring employee/patient satisfaction, intentions to leave, or burnout, then these would be considered interval scales. The interpretation of an interval scale provides context around higher or lower values, but someone rating burnout on a 1 to 5 scale as a 4 does not mean that this person is burnt out at a rate two times higher than someone rating a 2. This is where the last scale of measurement comes in, which is known as a *ratio scale*. It has the same properties as an interval scale but does have the presence of a true 0. A *true 0* means that there is a complete absence of the variable of interest. It also means you can make comparisons about values on the scale. An example of a ratio scale would be age or weight. For example, someone who is 40 years old is twice as old as someone who is 20 years old. This type of comparison between measures on a scale can *only* occur on a ratio scale.

Why Is It Important to Know What Type of Data I'm Collecting?

Scales of measurement dictate the statistical analyses that can be conducted. Recall that we broke down the types of variables that can be collected into four. Two of them are qualitative scales (nominal and ordinal) and the other two are quantitative scales (interval and ratio). Different statistical techniques are used depending on whether the data is quantitative or qualitative. Additionally, selecting the wrong statistical test for an analysis may result in the wrong outcome. Sometimes it's possible that the scale of measurement is hidden based on some additional analysis you conducted on the variable. Consider an example of a research study examining the impact of a program aimed at reducing the readmission rate for patients. Let's say that the study found a significant difference between the readmission rate at time A, which was 27%, compared to time B, which was 15%. It is critically important to know what scale of measurement a readmission rate is. To break it down further, readmission rates range from 0 to 100%. A readmission rate of 30% is twice that of a 15% readmission rate. You can also calculate an average readmission rate as well as the standard deviation. A 0% readmission rate means that no one was readmitted. Given this information and what was stated earlier regarding a ratio scale of measurement, this interpretation fits, so you may be inclined to say that readmission rates are ratio scales because there are quantitative properties and a true 0. That would be wrong, and here's why. When you are determining what the scale of measurement for a variable is, you need to focus on how that variable is being measured. Readmission rate is a calculated value, which is how we got to a percentage. Now ask yourself, how was the readmission rate calculated? It is based on the total number of patients who were readmitted divided by the total number of patients being studied. Therefore, the actual variable being measured is not really the readmission rate, but rather readmissions. What is the outcome of a readmission? A patient is either readmitted or not. This means that the readmission variable is measured on a nominal scale. A 1 was assigned to patients who were readmitted, and a 0 was assigned to patients who were not readmitted. Sometimes with variables we convert them to other measures that have meaning and context. In this case, we took all the 1s and 0s for readmitted and nonreadmitted patients and converted them to a percentage to interpret the variable.

Testing an Independent Variable

At this point you likely have already determined what intervention, phenomenon, or manipulation from the norm your research question aims to investigate. It is now time to determine how your intervention is carried out. Some interventions are actively implemented (e.g., nursing orientation class or new clinical practice guidelines), while others passively occur without any manipulation by the research team (e.g., inpatient ICU stay). The intervention phase requires careful planning to ensure consistency and reduction of potential influences that can skew your results. Here are some helpful strategies:

1) **Determine your intervention team and timeline:** As with sample recruiting, delivering an intervention is time consuming. Create realistic goals when determining how much time is needed. Team availability and willingness to commit to the study's purpose are important to completing a study. Create a schedule that meets realistic goals of data collection (e.g., four physicians will be interviewed each week until the intended sample size is met).

2) **Intervention team training:** Team meetings and trainings prior to initiating an intervention are extremely useful. Trainings should include a designated time for questions, demonstration, and reflection to avoid potential problems during data collection. They also allow the team to agree on a time frame for meeting goals.

3) **Use an intervention checklist:** A step-wise protocol that maps out exactly what is being done helps ensure that your sample is receiving a consistent intervention across all participants. Let's look at an example:

   A nurse is investigating the impact of a new topical cream that reduces discomfort during vaccine administration. Her checklist includes infection control precautions (e.g., handwashing and applying gloves) and lists the standard practice policy when cleaning the skin. She applies a numbing agent to the skin and waits 10 minutes prior to injecting the vaccine based on the recommended time frame of the topical anesthetic. The nurse records the time of the topical application and the time of the injection. She applies a band aid and immediately asks the patient to rate his discomfort on a scale from 1 to 10. The nurse records the score. If she had not included the 10-minute wait time and one of her team members waits only two minutes prior to injection, the pain or discomfort for the patient can vary. In addition, if the nurse waits to ask the patient about his discomfort level until the end of the visit and not immediately following the injection, the scores could potentially vary as well and would not be a reliable measure of determining if the topical cream reduces discomfort.

4) **Intervention timing:** During data collection, carefully consider appropriate timing that may or may not be crucial to your research question. Is the timing of your intervention ethical? Does the study interfere with patient care that can compromise a patient's outcomes? Does the timing of the data collection influence the phenomenon you are measuring? Example:

   If you aim to survey registered nurses about job-related fatigue, consider the differences in self-report responses at the beginning versus the end of a 12-hour shift.

5) **Data collection and handling:** You must follow your organization's policies when handling patient or staff information. We discuss the protection of human subjects and related policies later in the chapter. Start by creating a systematic method that organizes your data and makes it easy to follow for data analysis later on. When collecting quantitative data (empirical data), the use of spreadsheets and checklists with clear headings are helpful to keep track of data. Avoid abbreviations and vague terms that may be misinterpreted later on when analyzing your variables. When collecting qualitative data, note-taking and journals are helpful to map the collection process and any pitfalls that may have occurred. All data should be appropriately stored in a secure location (e.g., locked file cabinet in the investigator's office) or on a password-protected secure computer that is only accessible to the research team.

I Noticed That There Is Not an Exact Tool Out There to Measure What I Want. Can I Create My Own?

The most important part of the research process is to ensure that your research takes into consideration validity and reliability. Simply put, *validity* is the accuracy of your process/results, and *reliability* is the consistency of your process/results. These are two concepts that are extremely technical and have the ability to influence the results and conclusions you draw from your research. Every methodological decision you make will create additional issues that you must deal with.

Understanding validity and reliability is challenging, and we don't expect you to know everything about them in detail, but we do expect that you can make the appropriate decisions to strengthen your research design and achieve the desired results you are looking for. To illustrate how validity and reliability work, let's start with an example using a scale. When determining how to apply validity and reliability, you must think about the purpose of the instrument you are using to collect data. Validity cares about the result and how accurate it is, and reliability cares about the process. In the instance of a scale, validity would want to know if the result of the scale is accurate, and reliability would want to know that the process used to arrive at the result was consistent. The validity question would be, "Was the weight provided by the scale accurate for today, tomorrow, and every time I step on the scale?" The reliability question would be, "Does the scale always provide a value when I step on it?" This is important because when comparing and contrasting validity and reliability, it's very easy to say,

HINT!

Laminated checklists and pocket guides are beneficial, especially if the intervention is being carried out over an extended period of time and if your interventionist needs reminders of the steps while conducting the study.

"The scale is wrong because it didn't give me the right value." Let's dissect this last statement and ask why.

A scale is designed to weigh stuff. Is the scale always weighing stuff? If the answer to that question is yes, then it is reliably or consistently doing what it was designed to do. It was designed to weigh stuff. You wouldn't expect a scale to give you a temperature because it wasn't designed for that. The validity aspect is whether the result you get from the scale is accurate. If it is not accurate, then it is not valid. This leads to the relationship between validity and reliability. There are two conditions for this relationship:

1) Reliability is a necessary but not sufficient condition for validity.
2) Reliability is the upper limit to validity.

So, what do these mean? In the first statement, reliability is necessary to establish validity, but just because an instrument is reliable does not automatically mean it is valid. In using the scale example, let's say that every time you step on the scale it tells you that you are 5 or 10 pounds lighter. In this case it is reliably or consistently giving you your weight, but it is not accurate or valid. In the second statement, this means that the validity of your instrument is affected by its reliability. Both the reliability and the validity coefficients range from 0 to 1, with 1 being perfectly valid or reliable and 0 being neither valid nor reliable. The minimally acceptable reliability coefficient is traditionally around 0.7 (Cronbach, 1951). This means that with a reliability coefficient of 0.7, the validity cannot be higher than 0.7. In other words, there will always be some degree of error associated with an instrument, especially when measuring human behavior. We can make one guarantee with these two concepts: You can have an instrument that may be reliable and not valid, but it is impossible to have an instrument that is valid and not reliable. Once an instrument is determined to be valid it must always be reliable, but this relationship is not always perfect, as an acceptable reliability coefficient is above 0.7.

Reliability

Reliability generally revolves around five goals, purposes, or types. There are multiple techniques used to determine the reliability of an instrument. The most common form is *Cronbach's alpha*, which may be referred to as internal consistency or coefficient alpha. The majority of researchers report Cronbach's alpha in applied settings (Edwards et al., 2003), and it is the most widely reported form of reliability (Hogan et al., 2000; Rogers et al., 2002). Cronbach's alpha determines the extent to which the measures on your instrument actually measure what they are intended to measure.

Think of it this way: If you are administering a survey to patients that assesses their satisfaction or dissatisfaction with their hospital experience, then would you ask them only one question? You may actually ask them the question, "Overall, how satisfied or dissatisfied are you with your recent hospital stay?" and you will get an answer to that question. What you have to ask yourself is, how helpful would the results to that question be for making changes? The answer is not helpful. You would need to ask multiple questions to assess their hospital experience. You may want to ask about their room, the noise level, responses to call lights, their encounter with a physician or nurse, their experience with a mid-level provider, and how their pain was controlled. There are many questions that address the overall hospital experience, and the purpose of Cronbach's alpha would be to measure whether all the questions related to hospital experience actually measure hospital experience. The reliability of the instrument is the first step in understanding whether you have the ability to consistently collect information. If you cannot consistently gather information, then you would have no way of knowing if the results are accurate.

Validity

Once an instrument is determined to be reliable, then you want to ensure that it is accurate. The same is true when you design your research study. You want to ensure that the chosen design is valid. Think about this statement for a minute. What if I told you that I could tell you everything that will go wrong with your research *before* you even begin to collect data? To put it in a clinical perspective, wouldn't it be nice to know everything that could go wrong with a patient before you see that patient? You might be thinking that this is an impossible feat, but we can assure you that knowing the concept of validity can help you fix anything that can go wrong with your research before even collecting data. Now the caveat to this is that no research is perfect, and any decision you make will affect another part of the design. So, in other words, no research is perfect, which is why guidelines have been developed to determine what is acceptable. Recall that for reliability it is generally acceptable to have a coefficient of 0.7 or greater, and a power level is generally acceptable at 0.8 or above. For a decision to be significant, the *p-value* or significance level can be below 0.05, 0.01, or 0.001, which corresponds to a 95%, 99%, or 99.9% chance of being correct. There is always a chance something could go wrong, but it is your job as a researcher to try to prepare accordingly to avoid as many potential issues as possible.

There are four main types of validity: internal, external, statistical conclusion, and construct. Each of these types has threats or issues that affect the results. In total, there are 35 different threats to the validity of your study. This doesn't include the additive or interactive effect of threats, which means that some threats can act together to create a new type of threat to the results. Now you might be thinking, with everything that can go wrong, how can I do it right? The best offense is a good defense. Knowing all the threats and how to reduce them is your best defense, but don't get discouraged that you can't fix everything.

Going into detail on the nuances of validity and reliability is beyond the scope of this chapter. Readers who are interested in a more detailed explanation of validity and reliability should consult Picardi and Masick (2013) for more thorough explanations.

Can I Write My Own Survey Questions?

It's best to use a validated instrument, because writing survey items is an art. A lot of things can go wrong with writing a survey item, so it's best left to the experts. For example, asking a question like, "How satisfied are you with your career as nurse?" may seem like a straightforward and simple question, but it is not. Framing the question with "how satisfied" is a leading question. You are in fact leading a participant to believe they cannot be dissatisfied. This is also a vague question. If you are in fact rating your satisfaction with your career as a nurse, then what aspect of it are you rating? I bet if you asked five different nurses this question, they would all have different reasons for what makes them satisfied. This is extremely problematic because not everyone is interpreting the question exactly the same way. This also gets at the concept of an operational definition. There are multiple levels to most constructs, and writing your own questions limits the definition to how you interpret the construct, which may not be fully captured in one or two or 10 questions. A valid and reliable tool will ensure that everyone responds to the same question in the same way every time. A slightly better question than the one originally proposed could be, "How satisfied or dissatisfied are you with advancing your career as a nurse?"

Data Analysis Plan

I'm Not Familiar With Statistics. How Will I Analyze This Data?

Now that you've finished your data collection and made it through the process of conducting your own research, the next phase is analyzing the data. We do not expect you to become an expert in statistical analysis, but rather we want to equip you with the knowledge to have the conversation with a statistician and facilitate the process of drawing conclusions from your results.

Start with a few preliminary steps to immerse yourself in your data and determine what question you want to answer. *Simple descriptive statistics* are summaries about your sample and data. Start by identifying how you will divide your data (e.g., Yes versus No). Next, total the number of participants in each category (e.g., Male versus Female). *Frequency* is the number of participants in any given variable. You may choose to describe your data as a percentage (number of individuals with a specified response divided by the total sample size). An example of percentages would include: *40% of the sample reported greater than five years of clinical experience.* If you are using a survey instrument, refer to the instrument's instructions on how to interpret the scores. If your survey uses a total score, calculate the mean score of your total sample or divide by separate groups (e.g., those who received an intervention versus those who did not). To calculate the *mean* response of your sample, add all individual scores and divide by the total sample size.

What Is a Significance Level?

For some of your studies, you may want to test whether there is a significant difference between groups. It is important to solidify what you will be testing. The way in which you aggregate your data will determine what statistical tests you will conduct.

Comparing Groups

Your comparison may be within-groups or between-groups. *Within-group comparisons* generally investigate the differences between members within the same group. For example, if your targeted sample includes post-CABG patients over the age of 75, you can compare the outcomes between each patient within one group. On the other hand, *between-group comparisons* involve more than one group whose members may or may not have had the same intervention. For example, a nurse interested in determining the most effective discharge instructions to reduce post-hospitalization infection in patients with surgical wounds may implement an educational class in one group and a take-home pamphlet in a second group. A comparison would be made between those groups to determine if there was a difference in infection rates. Another comparison may include a *case-control group* where an intervention or some type of manipulation from the norm is implemented in one group (intervention group) and compared to a group that does not receive any intervention (control group). For example, a nursing researcher is interested in investigating how to reduce readmission rates of patients with congestive heart failure. The intervention group receives a post-discharge phone call to answer any questions the patients have regarding their plan of care. The control group does not receive a phone call. The outcomes—in this case, readmission rates—are compared.

Once you have determined which data to compare, you are ready to perform hypothesis testing. If you have never done hypothesis testing, we advise that you consult with a PhD-prepared researcher or biostatistician, whom you can find through your research council or relevant research departments. A few rules of thumb exist. If you are comparing two groups, the statistical test to perform is called a *t-test*. If you are comparing three or more groups, you will perform a test called *ANOVA*. These tests can be performed using statistical software (e.g., SPSS) that is accessible via your research department.

When Data Analysis Is Complete, How Will I Interpret the Findings?

Once you determine the statistical test, you need to figure out whether it is statistically significant. One caveat is the difference between statistical significance and clinical significance. Any test may result in an outcome that is statistically significant but not clinically significant or vice versa. The statistic you review to determine significance is the *p-value*, where the acceptable levels of significance are less than 0.05, 0.01, or 0.001. These values correspond to the probability or chance of finding significance. A p-value set at 0.05 means that there is a 95% chance of finding significance, a p-value of 0.01 means there is a 99% chance of finding significance, and 0.001 is a 99.9% chance of finding significance.

What If I Want to Interview Participants Instead of Using Surveys?

Some studies aim to capture the lived experience of a phenomenon or concept. In this case you may choose to perform one-on-one interviews or focus groups, called *qualitative research*. Several resources are available to guide you in conducting rigorous qualitative methodology and analyzing your data (Sandelowski, 1995). Start by defining your phenomenon clearly and using a theoretical framework to build your interview questions. The questions you ask during the interview should be open-ended to allow the interviewee to tell a story rather than simply answering yes or no. Prompts may be used, such as, "Tell me more" or, "Can you give me an example?" Interviews should be audio-recorded for review and analysis. There is a stepwise approach to analyzing qualitative data. Transcripts can be used to identify key components, dimensions, or emerging information. Two or more researchers should independently analyze the data and reach consensus about what information is emerging from the data. The goal is to identify emergent themes (*inductive analysis*) or to explore a specific theoretical model (*deductive analysis*). A third researcher can be used to resolve any discrepancies during the analysis. First, each researcher will "code" the data by identifying keywords or phrases. Next, through consensus you will group the codes into categories. Finally, determine which categories are related and group them into overarching themes or prespecified dimensions of your theoretical model.

How Many People Should I Interview?

The general rule of thumb is that you continue to interview until you reach *data saturation*, or when no new information is emerging. To reach saturation, you should interview and analyze data concurrently. By doing so, you can adjust your interview guide to further explore emergent themes. As you can imagine, broad research questions will require many more interviews compared to a specific question. Therefore, keep your timeline and resources in mind when refining your research question.

Summary

Conducting research is similar to asking the questions why, who, where, when, what, and how. The why is traditionally what led you to the present situation. You identified an issue that you want to solve, found literature support that your idea is worth pursuing, and found stakeholders who have an interest in what you want to do. With careful planning, conducting research is feasible and rewarding and can advance the scientific community by providing new or innovative approaches to solving everyday problems. Whether you are a seasoned researcher or brand-new to the concept of research, it can be overwhelming because there is no one way to conduct research. There are multiple paths to achieve the same result, but you must ensure that your research is as rigorous as you can make it to achieve the desired outcomes. There will always be obstacles that get in the way (time, resources, data availability, etc.) and prevent you from doing exactly what you want to do. However, knowing that there are multiple research designs, different hypotheses, and various ways of collecting data means that no matter what obstacle you are presented with, there is a way to overcome it to answer your question.

Our last piece of advice is not to be discouraged by what results you find or don't find. Research is meant to be cyclical in nature, and there is as much to be learned from what didn't work as from what did. The purpose of doing research is to be innovative and see your idea evolve into something that can be studied. As we have told our students in the past, look at the question you started with compared to the one you ended with and see if they are the same. As humans, we learn and grow from our experiences. These experiences come in the form of news articles, journals, our bosses, our peers, and our own personal journey to change something that we believe can be done differently. It is expected that the journey you start may be different from the end, and that's OK, because doing research is like driving down a curved roadway with lots of obstacles in the way. The point is, you'll never know what you can accomplish unless you start with an idea and execute it.

Review Questions

1. What name is given to the degree to which a measure assesses what it is supposed to measure (integrity of a measure)?
    A. Reliability
    B. Validity
    C. Statistical significance
    D. Clinical significance

    Answer: B. Validity is defined as the accuracy of a measure and is used to determine whether or not an instrument or tool was supposed to measure a variable of interest.

2. A nurse researcher is conducting a study in which one group of patients receives an educational brochure and a second group of patients does not. The research design described is a:
    A. Qualitative study
    B. Randomized clinical trial
    C. Pretest/posttest
    D. Case-control

    Answer: D. Case-Control is a type of research study in which one group receives an intervention and another group serves as a control where they do not receive the intervention.

3. Patients in a sample are asked to complete a satisfaction survey with a response scale from 1 (completed dissatisfied) to 5 (completely satisfied). What level of measurement does this describe?
    A. Nominal
    B. Ordinal
    C. Interval
    D. Ratio

    Answer: C. Interval is the most common Likert-type scale that measures a range of values with equal intervals between them.

4. You are conducting a retrospective descriptive study utilizing hospital claims data with only quality metrics and are not planning on collecting any personal health information (PHI). You would be submitting an IRB application for a(an)

   A. Full board review

   B. Expedited review

   C. Exempt study

   D. No IRB is necessary

Answer: C. Exempt study because the type of study being done does not collect any patient identifiers and the purpose is for assessing quality within your own organization.

5. You are analyzing a research study that compares the patient outcomes of a sepsis treatment protocol to patients who received the current protocol to determine if the new protocol results in improved outcomes. For the groups, you are comparing:

   A. Within-groups

   B. Cohort groups

   C. Between-groups

   D. Case-control groups

Answer: C. Between-groups is done when you are analyzing two different groups and they only are exposed to one treatment.

References

Cronbach, L. J. (1951). Coefficient alpha and the internal structure of tests. *Psychometrika, 16*(3), 297–334.

Edwards, J. E., Scott, J. C., & Raju, N. S. (2003). *The Human resources program-evaluation handbook.* Sage Publications.

Hogan, T. P., Benjamin, A., & Brezinski, K. L. (2000). Reliability methods: A note on the frequency of use of various types. *Educational and Psychological Measurement, 60*(4), 523–531.

Picardi, C.A., & Masick, K.D. (2013). *Designing and conducting research with a real-world focus.* Sage Publications. Thousand Oaks: CA.

Rogers, W. N., Schmitt, N., & Mullins, M. E. (2002). Correction for unreliability of multifactor measures: Comparison of alpha and parallel forms approaches. *Organizational Research Methods, 5*(2), 184–199.

Sandelowski, M. (1995). Qualitative analysis: What it is and how to begin. *Research in Nursing & Health, 18*(4), 371–375.

PEACE MODEL

P

PROBLEM IDENTIFICATION
Formulate the clinical question (**PICO**):
- **P** | Patient Population
- **I** | Intervention
- **C** | Comparison of Intervention
- **O** | Outcome

E

EVIDENCE REVIEW
Review evidence relevant to your clinical question by searching databases.

A

APPRAISE EVIDENCE
Appraise the evidence that appears highest in the hierarchy of scientific evidence for its quality and applicability to practice.

C

CHANGE PRACTICE OR CONDUCT RESEARCH
If evidence is sufficient, embark on improvement project to address practice change.

If evidence is insufficient to warrant practice change, conduct research.

E

EVALUATE AND DISSEMINATE FINDINGS
Evaluate the impact of the implemented practice change and research results.

Disseminate findings through publication, oral, and poster presentations.

7

EVALUATION

–Kenrick D. Cato, PhD, RN, CPHIMS, FAAN
Michele P. Holskey, DNP, RN, NEA-BC

KEYWORDS | PHRASES

outcomes evaluation, outcome measures, process measures,
SQUIRE guidelines, cost analysis

CHAPTER OBJECTIVES

After studying this chapter, learners will be able to:

1. Explain the role of evaluation in the evidence-based project life cycle.

2. Identify the difference between process measures and outcome measures.

3. Describe the importance of planning in the evaluation step of the PEACE model.

Introduction

This chapter includes information about project evaluation related to implementation of the PEACE model. The following scenario is designed to highlight issues that may arise when not planning adequately for evaluation of your evidence-based practice (EBP) project:

> A group of nurses on the Unit Quality Committee decide to conduct a project to improve patient outcomes on their unit. They agree to implement an early mobilization protocol that a nurse learned about at a national professional nursing organization conference. The nurses on the committee took the time to research the literature about the benefits of early mobilization and provided a summary of the literature to their nurse

manager. The nurse manager successfully advocates for the nurses using the literature review summary to get approval from her superiors.

With that green light the nurses implement the EBP project and, because they know data will be required, they decide to administer a satisfaction survey to patients upon discharge. This project is conducted for six months, and while it takes a lot of work to successfully perform the data collection, the nurses get the job done. Then the committee members take another six months to analyze the survey results and present the findings to the nurse leaders.

On presentation day the nurses are excited because they notice a difference in patient outcomes after the project was implemented. The nurses report that patients were satisfied with their progress and that patient length of stay seemed shorter after early mobilization was implemented. After the committee gives their presentation to their CNO, she has a few questions. First, she wants to know about the project steps. How did the nurses decide what to evaluate in the project? How was the survey created and validated? Second, she wants to know how patient experience and length of stay were affected by the project, because patient experience and stay duration have real economic value. Finally, the CNO wants to know the nurses' plans to disseminate their findings. This work should be shared across the organization and could serve as a burning question for future nursing research.

The nurses on the committee did their best to answer all these questions but leave the talk deflated, yet curious. Honestly, they had not considered the things that the CNO asked them. However, the conversation with the CNO sparked their interest for answering the "so what" questions that are essential when evaluating the effectiveness of changes in nursing practice based on evidence. The nurses wondered: (1) Was their evaluation appropriate? (2) Are their findings really meaningful? (3) What should they do next, because the findings may not have any worth.

I hope you never find yourself in this situation. The most important takeaway from this chapter is plan, plan, plan. Use the knowledge that we give you to plan your project so that you will not have major regrets after a lot of time and hard work.

Evaluation of Outcomes

Research has shown that EBP improves patient safety, quality of care, and health outcomes (Harper et al., 2017). For this reason, you might find yourself conducting your own EBP project. One of the critical and often challenging parts of any project is deciding how to measure its success. The process of measuring success is called *evaluation*.

EBP Evaluation

EBP evaluation should be a planned part of the whole project life cycle rather than an afterthought. In other words, you do not want to find yourself unable to answer the "so what?" question after completing a project and saying, "Well, what can I measure to show that it worked?"

Broadly speaking, there are two types of planned EBP project evaluations of improvement: process and outcome measures. *Process measures* indicate what the clinician did in giving and receiving care to maintain or improve health. Examples of process measures are mostly compliance processes that influence outcomes, such as the number or percentage of patients evaluated or the number of caregivers who received education. *Outcome measures* are considered the gold standard of measurement and include impacts of improvements on people and organizations often dealing with health and well-being. Examples of outcome or performance measures are patient satisfaction, infection rates, mortality, length of stay, adverse events, blood pressures, and cost savings. When nurses conduct research and quality improvement interventions, they must plan in advance the measures to be carefully collected and accurately analyzed to determine the significance of their work. Then nurses can evaluate the result and success (or lack thereof) of the changes and implications for next steps in the EBP process.

When selecting the appropriate outcome measures, you need to identify benchmarks and best practices for measuring, examining, and comparing the impacts of your project. For example, if you are planning to reduce healthcare-associated infection rates, you would compare your organization infection rates to like organizations, specifically at the unit level when possible. Top-performing organizations exceed national benchmarks, which are typically a statistic, such as mean infection rates (per 1,000 central line days, for example, when comparing central line–associated bloodstream infections). When your unit experiences a central line infection, nurses are obligated to compare their practices to benchmarks, best practices, national guidelines, and regulatory recommendations to improve quality outcomes and safe nursing care.

When deciding how to evaluate your EBP intervention, there are a few very important questions that you should ask:

- **Are the concepts I want to measure measurable?** This may seem like an obvious question. However, most clinical environments have limited resources. For example, if you want to evaluate patients' weight loss, consistent weighing must happen. There are a number of related questions that should be asked. Does that fit into the current workflow? Are individuals trained to consistently and effectively make the assessments?

- **Do I have a valid instrument to perform the measurement?** The tool that is used to assess weight loss is easy. It is a scale. But what if you wanted to measure communication between nurses and doctors? Often, nurses do their best to create a tool for these types of measurements. But you should know that tool development is a science all to itself. Also, if there is something you want to measure, a scientist has probably created an already validated tool to measure that concept. So instead of spending the late nights creating your own survey, you should look into the literature and find an already validated tool to measure interdisciplinary communication.

- **Do I have a systematic method to maintain and sustain change?** The goal of EBP projects is to bring evidence into your practice that will improve patient and clinician outcomes. To accomplish this, the practice change must be sustainable. There are many strategies for sustaining change, such as leadership champions, management support, ongoing professional development, integration of evidence-based interventions in policies and procedures, and engaging interprofessionals in the change (Melnyk & Fineout-Overholt, 2019). The structured Plan Do Study Act (PDSA) cycle will ensure that the EBP life cycle is sustainable. In PDSA, nurses plan small tests of change, including decisions about what data are collected, and implement the changes. As part of the cycle, nurses analyze data and identify what worked and what did not work. Next, nurses refine the change and repeat the cycle to determine its impact on the desired outcome. Nurses make the best-informed decisions about sustained changes to nursing practice when they combine findings from evidence-based quality improvement projects and evidence from research.

Research Evaluation

The evaluation of research is equally important as the evaluation of evidence-based quality improvement projects. Research should be conducted to generate new knowledge (Hulley, 2013). For research, evaluation reflects the research question and actual research design. Research design can be complex; however, the main issue is how involved you want to get in measurement, with observational studies being more passive than experimental clinical trials, where intervention effects are rigorously evaluated. For example, healthcare organizations attempt to measure nurse satisfaction at frequent intervals to reduce turnover and improve satisfaction. When considering a study investigating drivers of nurse engagement, nurse leaders may administer a validated tool to survey nurses, such as nurses in an inpatient psychiatric hospital. Using a cross-sectional study design, nurse leaders could compare the results to national benchmarks and describe the findings based on that time period.

Table 7.1 explains the characteristics of research design and evaluation by applying different approaches to a hypothetical study focused on determining the levels of engagement among psychiatric nurses.

Table 7.1 | **Example of Nursing Research Design on Drivers of Engagement Among Psychiatric Nurses**

Research Design Type	Research Focus	Hypothetical Example
Observational Designs		
Cohort study, prospective	One group is identified, and the same group is followed over time and compared to a different group of people	Nurse researcher measures drivers of engagement among nurses in an inpatient psychiatric hospital at the beginning of the study and then measures at regular intervals to determine if the drivers changed over time.
Case-control or retrospective study	Two groups (cases) are selected and compared based on presence or absence of an outcome	Nurse researcher measures nurses who work in a psychiatric inpatient setting and compares them with nurses who work in a different practice environment, such as rehabilitation nurses.
Cross-sectional study	One group is measured at one point in time or time interval	Nurse researcher obtains assessments of current drivers of engagement among nurses in an inpatient psychiatric hospital and describes the findings based on that time period.
Experimental Clinical Trial Design		
Randomized control trial	A random process is used to assign people to an experimental or a control group	Nurse researcher randomly assigns people to receive CBD or a placebo and then follows both groups for a specified time period to measure chronic pain in each group.

SQUIRE Guidelines

As an alternative to research design, if you are conducting an EBP project or quality improvement project, your goal should be to design a project and disseminate your findings about the contributions you have made for improved patient, organization, and community outcomes. The primary mode of dissemination is through peer-reviewed publication. To successfully publish, you must ensure that your manuscript is of high quality. In the 1990s, researchers and editors began to create guidelines to improve the quality of EBP and quality articles (Davidoff et al., 2008). SQUIRE stands for Standards for QUality Improvement Reporting Excellence. The SQUIRE guidelines were developed to standardize the reporting of quality and EBP findings for purposes of improving the quality, safety, and value of healthcare (Ogrinc et al., 2016). These guidelines (http://www.squire-statement. org/) are actually a checklist of how to report new knowledge and include suggested elements for dissemination (Davidoff et al., 2008).

Over time, the SQUIRE guidelines have evolved to serve a few purposes. First, SQUIRE is the industry standard, with publishers expecting that authors will follow the guidelines for EBP and quality articles. Second, people now use SQUIRE as a project planning tool to understand what components will be necessary for successful completion. Finally, you can use the SQUIRE guidelines to evaluate a project. For example, you can go to the SQUIRE website, print out the checklist, and compare it to your manuscript to see if you fulfilled all the required criteria.

Cost as a Dimension of EBP

EBP is the standard for most high-performing healthcare settings. In nursing, the highly sought-after American Nurses Credentialing Center's Magnet Recognition Program® designation places EBP at the center of nursing excellence (Anderson et al., 2018). However, when pursuing practice change, nurses need to advocate for and justify the required organizational commitment. In our current regulatory and consumer-influenced environment, healthcare organizations should recognize that poor patient, organizational, and community outcomes are detrimental to the financial bottom line (Melnyk et al., 2018). The demonstration of the cost benefit of a project can be an important component of not only obtaining but also justifying practice change to improve the performance of an organization (Wurmser, 2009). While there is much support in the literature for the improvement of quality and cost outcomes when clinical practice is guided by the latest evidence (Mackey &

Bassendowski, 2017), the procurement of precious resources can still be challenging for nurses. Therefore, to overcome business as usual, clinical nurses and their leaders must align resource needs with the strategic initiatives of the organization, which requires cost evaluation as a crucial element of any project. When nurses demonstrate that they have evaluated the cost impact and savings associated with an EBP project, they strengthen their partnership with financial stakeholders and leaders. By planning and utilizing effective tools of cost analysis to demonstrate that EBP is a good investment, you can support its implementation sustainability by ensuring that the project is clinically effective, efficient, and financially sound (Iribarren et al., 2017).

Cost Considerations

To implement a viable EBP project, you must understand what is involved from a cost perspective. First, what are the costs involved in establishing an effective program? Costs that you should consider include those associated with 1) establishing the EBP infrastructure, 2) performing required staff education, and 3) implementing the change in practice. Transformational nurse leaders can serve as mentors to frontline nurses to identify costs and make recommendations for resource allocations.

Infrastructure Costs

Infrastructure costs can be thought of as resource costs associated with a project. Infrastructure is a general category that includes physical items like a new machine as well an individual time or effort, which is usually measured by portions of a person's salary. Nurses often consider costs associated with supplies, equipment, and possibly new staffing models required for a project. However, one should not forget to assess the increased or new use of existing resources. For example, nurses should consider how much increased committee participation, project meeting, and individual planning time will be incurred. Be sure to include resources outside of your department, and take advantage of the interprofessional team, such as materials management, facility operations, and human resource managers, to ensure an inclusive list of infrastructure costs.

Staff Education Costs

In addition to infrastructure, there will be education costs. Introduction of new processes is less likely to succeed without adequate staff education. For your project, you should take the time to assess all the resources (including who will provide the education) required to teach a change in practice. With EBP education, there are a few points to consider that will influence the cost. First, how best can the education fit into clinical workflow? For example, if all shifts need the training, will the night shift have to come in early or stay late? In that case, overtime costs must be factored into the total costs associated with a project. Often, organizations create online learning modules to optimize accessibility. While these electronic education offerings increase learner flexibility, they are often costly to create and implement.

Implementation Costs

After you have considered the infrastructure and education, there are implementation costs. These are the costs that are associated with changes that are needed to have the new practice occur day in and day out. Your goal is to effect evidence-based clinical change. Therefore, you should consider what will be necessary to sustain your implementation over time. In the long term, successful implementation often requires a number of actions, including refresher and new staff education, equipment maintenance and replacement, and eventual project outcome evaluation. Ideally, all the outlined tasks should occur, but resource limitation will influence what you can realistically accomplish; tradeoff and compromises will be needed. This is where a serious consideration of feasibility and cost should be performed. It is only through a careful assessment of the costs and benefits that you will identify a sustainable EBP implementation that will achieve your clinical and financial goals.

Overview of Tools for Economic Evaluation

While searching the literature, you may find many articles that claim to perform an economic evaluation; however, few are able to deliver the analysis you need. There are a few required features of real economic evaluation that address the efficiencies, benefits, and return on investments. Overall, economic evaluations are a specific set of analysis methods that are designed to make decisions in different healthcare situations (Drummond et al., 2015). Regardless of the project topic, one question must be addressed: Are we sure that additional precious healthcare resources (for an intervention, practice change, equipment, or staffing) should or should not be spent in this way?

Well-constructed economic evaluations always have a few features. First, there are always inputs and outputs, which are usually described as costs and consequences for different courses of action. For example, a project could require the hiring of unit-level wound care nurses to help prevent and decrease pressure injuries. For this proposed project, the costs (what we have to give up) would be the money required for the additional nurses' salary, and the consequences (the expected benefits) would be improved patient outcomes related to pressure injuries. Second, economic evaluations are all about choices. Continuing with our example, we know that resources are limited, and nurse leaders are committed to balanced unit and organization budgets. Therefore, we can assume that the salary of the additional wound care nurses will require taking away money or saving costs in another area in the budget. These choices will have to be made based on known and measurable criteria. Third, economic evaluations usually compare different scenarios. Comparison is an important component. There could be multiple comparisons, like hiring a specialized wound care nurse, or comparing costs for training existing nurses as wound care champions. Also, an option in the scenario could be to do nothing and see the associated financial impact of that. In summary, you can think of economic evaluation as a set of steps to identify, measure, assign value to, and compare costs and consequences for different scenarios.

You might be wondering if all economic evaluations use the same techniques. The answer is no; there are a number of distinct approaches that depend on the types of costs and consequences of your specific project. This can best be demonstrated by the five different examples of economic evaluations discussed in the following sections.

Cost-Consequence Analysis

This technique is used to ignore costs. Instead, a series of outcome data (costs) is presented to allow individuals to evaluate the consequences.

Cost-Effectiveness Analysis

This method is used to understand new practices or strategies from a nonmonetary perspective. Imagine that you are thinking about the cost associated with a new intervention to improve outcomes for patients with complications of diabetes using lifestyle changes and medication versus just medication alone. In this example, nurses would compare the costs and consequences of medication alone versus lifestyle changes and medication to arrive at the most cost-effective interventions. The costs are usually modeled over a specified time horizon per year or over a lifetime. Also, for this approach the consequences are measured as an incremental cost-effectiveness ratio (ICER). Usually the ICER is expressed as cost per life years gained or costs per quality adjusted life year (QALY; Dick et al., 2015). For these analyses, life year gained or QALY serves as useful to determine between two or more interventions which intervention or practice change is meaningful from a life span perspective.

Cost-Minimization Analysis

This method is used to highlight the least expensive option that is under consideration. This approach compares the net costs of a process or intervention and assumes that each option has relatively similar outcomes. For example, when comparing the costs of three new syringe products that all have similar nurse safety and health outcomes, you would choose the less expensive option.

Cost-Utility Analysis

This approach compares different health outcomes. For this technique the QALY gained is used to compare each intervention. This multidimensional analysis is a closer measure of a person's well-being. For example, you might want to compare a patient's health outcome for an elective surgery versus pharmacological treatment.

Cost-Benefit Analysis

In comparison to a cost-utility analysis, this technique attempts to put a monetary value on health benefits or quality of life to compare interventions.

Summary

It is our hope that you now understand the importance of evaluation in the PEACE model. When planning your EBP projects, it is crucial that you take time to determine how you will evaluate the project. Beyond evaluation planning, we covered a number of important concepts. First, be sure you determine if you will be using process and outcome measures. Decide in advance which outcomes will be monitored to answer the "so what" question and ensure that nursing practice changes are aligned with the organization's strategic priorities and sustained over time. Second, consider how you may use cost analysis in your evaluation. Based on your thorough evaluation of practice changes and research results, you will apply research, conduct new research, consider new quality improvement projects, and disseminate findings and new knowledge (Tahan et al., 2016). Finally, the SQUIRE guidelines provide a useful checklist for all of the necessary components of your EBP project and prepare you for publishing the contributions you made to transforming nursing practice and healthcare outcomes.

Review Questions

1. **What is the most important part of evaluation?**

   Answer: The most important part of evaluation of research and EBP is planning in advance.

2. **What are the two types of measures that you would use to evaluate your EBP project?**

   Answer: Two types of measures for evaluating your EBP project are process measures and outcome measures, which need to be determined in advance of starting your project. Outcome measures will assist you to answer the "so what" question and ensure that nursing practice changes are aligned with the organization's strategic priorities.

3. **What are the five types of cost analysis?**

   Answer: The five types of cost analysis are cost-consequence analysis, cost-effectiveness analysis, cost-minimization analysis, cost-utility analysis, and cost-benefit analysis.

4. **How can you use the SQUIRE guidelines in your EBP work?**

   Answer: The SQUIRE guidelines include industry standards and publisher expectations for EBP and quality improvement articles. SQUIRE serves as a project planning tool and checklist that may be printed and compared to your manuscript to ensure that you fulfilled all the required criteria.

5. **When deciding how to evaluate your EBP intervention, what are some important considerations?**

   Answer: In addition to careful planning, key considerations for the evaluation of EBP are to ensure that the concepts you intend to measure are measurable, to use a valid instrument when performing the measurement, and to have a systematic method for maintaining and sustaining evidence-based changes in nursing practice.

References

Anderson, V. L., Johnston, A. N., Massey, D., & Bamford-Wade, A. (2018). Impact of MAGNET hospital designation on nursing culture: An integrative review. *Contemporary Nurse*, 54(4–5), 483–510.

Davidoff, F., Batalden, P., Stevens, D., Ogrinc, G., & Mooney, S. (2008). Publication guidelines for quality improvement in health care: Evolution of the SQUIRE project. *BMJ Quality & Safety, 17*(Suppl. 1), i3–i9.

Dick, A. W., Perencevich, E. N., Pogorzelska-Maziarz, M., Zwanziger, J., Larson, E. L., & Stone, P. W. (2015). A decade of investment in infection prevention: A cost-effectiveness analysis. *American Journal of Infection Control, 43*(1), 4–9.

Drummond, M. F., Sculpher, M. J., Claxton, K., Stoddart, G. L., & Torrance, G. W. (2015). *Methods for the economic evaluation of health care programmes*. Oxford University Press.

Harper, M. G., Gallagher-Ford, L., Warren, J. I., Troseth, M., Sinnott, L. T., & Thomas, B. K. (2017). Evidence-based practice and US healthcare outcomes: Findings from a national survey with nursing professional development practitioners. *Journal for Nurses in Professional Development, 33*(4), 170–179.

Hulley, S. B., Cummings, S. R., Browner, W. S., Grady, D., & Newman, T. B. (2013). *Designing clinical research* (4th ed.). Lippincott Williams & Wilkins.

Iribarren, S. J., Cato, K., Falzon, L., & Stone, P. W. (2017). What is the economic evidence for mHealth? A systematic review of economic evaluations of mHealth solutions. *PLoS ONE, 12*(2), e0170581.

Mackey, A., & Bassendowski, S. (2017). The history of evidence-based practice in nursing education and practice. *Journal of Professional Nursing, 33*(1), 51–55.

Melnyk, B. M., & Fineout-Overholt, E. (2019). *Evidence-based practice in nursing & healthcare: A guide to best practice* (4th ed.). Wolters Kluwer/Lippincott Williams & Wilkins.

Melnyk, B. M., Gallagher-Ford, L., Zellefrow, C., Tucker, S., Thomas, B., Sinnott, L. T., & Tan, A. (2018). The first US study on nurses' evidence-based practice competencies indicates major deficits that threaten healthcare quality, safety, and patient outcomes. *Worldviews on Evidence-Based Nursing, 15*(1), 16–25.

Ogrinc, G., Davies, L., Goodman, D., Batalden, P., Davidoff, F., & Stevens, D. (2016). SQUIRE 2.0 (Standards for QUality Improvement Reporting Excellence): Revised publication guidelines from a detailed consensus process. *BMJ Quality & Safety, 25*(12), 986–992.

Tahan, H. M., Rivera, R. R., Carter, E. J., Gallagher, K. A., Fitzpatrick, J. J., & Manzano, W. M. (2016). Evidence-based practice: The PEACE framework. *Nurse Leader, 14*(1), 57–61.

Wurmser, T. (2009). The financial case for EBP. *Nursing Management, 40*(2), 12–14.

PEACE MODEL

PROBLEM IDENTIFICATION

Formulate the clinical question (**PICO**):

P | Patient Population
I | Intervention
C | Comparison of Intervention
O | Outcome

EVIDENCE REVIEW

Review evidence relevant to your clinical question by searching databases.

APPRAISE EVIDENCE

Appraise the evidence that appears highest in the hierarchy of scientific evidence for its quality and applicability to practice.

CHANGE PRACTICE OR CONDUCT RESEARCH

If evidence is sufficient, embark on improvement project to address practice change.

If evidence is insufficient to warrant practice change, conduct research.

EVALUATE AND DISSEMINATE FINDINGS

Evaluate the impact of the implemented practice change and research results.

Disseminate findings through publication, oral, and poster presentations.

8

DISSEMINATE FINDINGS

–Kristine M. Kulage, MA, MPH | Reynaldo R. Rivera, DNP, RN, NEA-BC, FAAN

KEYWORDS | PHRASES

dissemination, disseminate findings, peer-reviewed publication, podium presentation, poster presentation, research findings, research studies

CHAPTER OBJECTIVES

After studying this chapter, learners will be able to:

1. Identify why research dissemination is important.
2. Describe the various ways to disseminate study findings.
3. Determine the appropriateness of dissemination of study findings.

Introduction

To advance the field of nursing, it is vital that nurses disseminate new knowledge. If colleagues do not know about their work, then change cannot occur. By disseminating study findings through articles in peer-reviewed journals and presentations at professional conferences, you can add to the body of knowledge in your area of expertise and contribute to improving patient care. There are several types of articles for disseminating your work; choosing the right article type is key to ensuring your work will be presented in the proper context to share your knowledge. The most common writing products in nursing are the case study, the clinical practice manuscript, the quality improvement manuscript, literature reviews (i.e., scoping, integrative, systematic, meta-analyses), and the research manuscript. One resource available for guided, step-by-step instructions for effective scholarly writing and dissemination from a nursing perspective is Oermann and Hays' *Writing for Publication in Nursing* (Oermann & Hays, 2018).

Disseminating Findings Through Peer-Reviewed Publications

Kulage and Larson (2016) provide five tips for increasing your writing productivity:

1. Set aside non-negotiable writing time.
2. Always write for your reader.
3. Show, don't tell.
4. Break big jobs into smaller tasks.
5. Stop writing when you know what you are going to write next (see Kulage and Larson [2016] for more details on these tips).

The importance of writing for your reader should be emphasized to ensure readers understand your message. It is imperative to avoid *jargon*—field-specific terminology and rhetoric familiar only to individuals in your field of expertise. Keep your readers in mind, or you risk losing them on the path to explaining your work and its impact. Put yourself in the position of your reader and ask, "What does this reader need to know to understand what I am writing?" This is also related to choosing the appropriate journal for your manuscript. You can be successful in writing for your reader by taking into account "Who is the audience for this journal?" and "Who is ultimately going to be reading this article—in other words, what does their experience, expertise, and knowledge profile look like?"

Choosing a Journal

There are several questions to answer while choosing an appropriate journal. These include:

- What are my goals?
- Who is my audience? Are they internal or external to the field? Are they practitioners, administrators, or policymakers?
- What is the scope of influence I am hoping my work has? Am I looking to simply disseminate information, or am I looking to invoke change in practice or policy?

Because the voice and tone of your manuscript will be driven by answers to these questions, choosing your journal should be your first step (Morton, 2013). Educate yourself on the journals you are considering; they all have a brief mission statement and identify their target audience and areas of interest. Consider contacting the editor in advance to assess the journal's level of interest in your topic.

If you are unfamiliar with journals in your area of expertise, the Directory of Nursing Journals of the International Academy of Nursing Editors (INANE) is a free online resource (https://nursingeditors.com/journals-directory/) that allows you to view nursing-related journals alphabetically or search the list by keywords. Journal entries include basic information such as the editor, publisher, sponsoring organization, a link to author guidelines, and a description of the mission. In addition, the INANE website (https://nursingeditors.com/) has a wealth of resources on editing, reviewing, and publishing your work; related professional organizations and conferences; and journal impact factors (for more information on the impact factor and how it may affect your journal choice, see Garfield, 2006). Before deciding on a journal, it is a good idea to read several articles in the journals you are considering. This will help you ascertain what types of articles are typically published.

Predatory Journals

When searching for a journal, avoid potential predatory journals. While Cobey and colleagues indicate that "there is currently no agreed upon definition of what constitutes a predatory journal" (Cobey et al., 2018, p. 3), librarian Jeffrey Beall coined the term *predatory journal* in 2012, referring to publishers that "publish counterfeit journals to exploit the open-access model in which the author pays" and remarked that such publishers were "dishonest and lack transparency" (Beall, 2012, p. 179; Cobey et al., 2018, p. 3). A recent scoping review presents a summary of characteristics found in predatory journals, including poor quality or deceptive: (1) journal operations, (2) articles, (3) editorial and peer-review processes, (4) communications, (5) processing charges, and (6) dissemination, indexing, and archiving services (Cobey et al., 2018). The recent increase in the number of predatory journals has prompted the creation of websites that list potential predatory journals. Beall's List of Predatory Journals and Publishers (https://beallslist.net/) not only presents an extensive list of potential predatory scholarly open-access publishers and their journals but also provides other links to and resources for related information such as questionable conferences and an evaluation tool for assessing whether a journal is predatory. Stop Predatory Journals (www.predatoryjournals.com) provides a list of thousands of possible predatory journals and links to their websites and allows the option for visitors to report potential new predatory journals. Use care when choosing the journal for your manuscript, and investigate its potential for being predatory if you are not already familiar with it before proceeding.

Scholarly Writing Basics

Scholarly writing is essentially scientific writing or technical writing. It is considered nonfiction and is not creative writing you would find in a novel. It is writing that informs, teaches, and explains. It is not storytelling, which has a goal of entertaining readers. Instead, you are explaining something but in a compelling way with a goal of informing and educating the reader. In creative writing, twists and turns in a story, such as surprise endings, keep readers interested. In scholarly writing you do not want to surprise readers. For example, in your abstract and introduction you will make promises to your reader about what you will be covering in your manuscript, and it is important to keep that promise and deliver on it to eliminate surprise and avoid confusion. In scholarly writing, you must be consistent in your terminology. Use exact words, choose them carefully, and be consistent. Be succinct and avoid wordiness. Your job in scholarly writing it to lay out a road map for your reader that is easy to follow, with headings and subheadings as signposts along the way. When writing for a professional journal, you will likely be faced with the challenge of limiting your writing to a specific length that is shorter than what you believe you need to explain your project or study. Being brief and precise has multiple advantages in scholarly writing and, in particular, writing for peer-reviewed journals.

Authorship and Author Order

Collaborative writing, a partnership with one or more scholars or coauthors who provide support for the content, writing, and editing of a paper, is common in academia. It can be a rewarding experience that can increase the chances that your manuscript is accepted for publication, particularly if the work is interdisciplinary in nature. It brings together input from multiple individuals with a wide array of expertise as compared to a single author writing in a silo. While the lead author holds primary responsibility for writing the manuscript, because the nature of research is also collaborative, each participant in the research project may be responsible for writing a section reflecting the work performed. However, collaborative writing can be a source of conflict, particularly when it comes to the topic of authorship and the order of authors. The International Committee of Medical Journal Editors (ICMJE) publishes the uniform requirements for manuscripts submitted to biomedical journals, which delineates how an individual can earn authorship on a manuscript (ICMJE, 2010). Most biomedical journals have adopted the ICMJE definition of authors; thus, it is good practice to follow this guidance when determining who has earned a spot as an author and who should just be acknowledged at the end of a manuscript. According to the ICMJE, all three of the following conditions must be met to earn authorship (ICMJE, 2010):

1. They substantially contributed to the conception and design or acquisition of data or analysis and interpretation of data in the paper.
2. They should have been part of drafting the article or revising it critically for important intellectual content.
3. They are one of the individuals who must give approval of the final version of the manuscript to be published.

Things are not as well-defined regarding the order of authors on a manuscript. Some journals provide guidance on this, but most do not. Author order is typically decided by the level of contribution. First authors usually led or performed most of the work of the study and held primary responsibility for drafting, revising, and finalizing the manuscript. Senior (i.e., last) authors often participated in planning the study and may have also helped conduct it, but their writing contributions are normally limited to reviewing and revising drafts of the manuscript and supervising the first author's writing. The order of the remaining authors can be determined by level of contribution to the study and the writing, or even alphabetically if all contributed equally. Baerlocher and colleagues (2007) provide additional guidance and recommendations on the meaning of author order in medical research.

Following Guidelines

To ensure clear and consistent presentation of written material, all journals provide a set of author guidelines that must be followed in manuscripts submitted for publication consideration. Guidelines include everything from general instructions on word limits, section headings, order of sections, presentation of tables and figures, and formatting of citations and references to fine details such as page margins, line spacing, font type and size, and text alignment. These guidelines are typically located in a section of the journal website called "Information for Authors" and may also be published in the hard copy of journal issues. Many guidelines for journals published in the nursing and healthcare fields follow an already well-established set of rules called a "style," such as the American Psychological Association (APA) style (www.apastyle.org) or the American Medical Association (AMA) style (www.amamanualofstyle.com), which dictate formatting, layout, and many other elements on how your manuscript must be constructed. Some journals specify guidelines that follow some elements of a specific style but provide other rules that may divert from that standard style. Because there are so many variations in the journal publishing world, authors must carefully read all author guidelines and adhere to them in preparing their manuscript. If a manuscript does not follow the guidelines, some journals may return them to the author for correction before they go out to reviewers. In some cases, editors may simply reject the manuscript outright. In other cases, if manuscripts are sent to reviewers formatted improperly, they may get a negative review, even if the content of the manuscript is strong. Making sure your manuscript is formatted properly from the beginning not only displays professionalism but also means less work for you at the copyediting and proofing phases if your manuscript is accepted for publication.

When writing a manuscript, one of the more challenging aspects is properly adding citations and keeping track of your list of references—and making sure they follow the journal guidelines. Use of reference management software that allows you to collect, organize, and use bibliographic references is strongly recommended, as manual maintenance of citations can be extremely time-consuming and ultimately fraught with errors. Three of the most popular reference management software programs are EndNote (www.endnote.com), Mendeley (www.mendeley.com), and Zotero (www.zotero.com). Cost and access should be considered when choosing your software. EndNote has more options (e.g., a desktop and online version) but has a license fee, while Mendeley and Zotero are online only but are free to use. Your institutional library may have a subscription to EndNote, making it freely available for you to download. If you need to share your reference lists with other authors or you work on your manuscript from different locations on multiple devices, an online option may be best. Importantly, all reference management software packages allow you to specify output styles for citations and reference lists according to journal guidelines, or tweak existing styles to make new, tailored ones if needed. In addition, these software programs interface with major bibliographic indices used to search for literature, such as PubMed (www.ncbi.nlm.nih.gov/pubmed) and Google Scholar (www.scholar.google.com), enabling you to import references seamlessly into your program and then your manuscript. Institutional libraries typically offer free tutorials on the use of these reference management software programs, but opportunities for independent training through websites or YouTube videos are also available.

Reviewing the Literature

Before writing a manuscript, it is crucial that you conduct a literature review. You will learn what previous work has been done on your topic and find out how your work is related to existing work. For example, it is very possible that similar work was published but in a different clinical setting (e.g., adult versus pediatric or medical-surgical versus emergency department). Importantly, your literature search will help you determine if your work contributes new knowledge, a key component to justify publication and dissemination of your study. Information from a review of the literature is typically presented in two places in a manuscript: the introduction and the discussion. In the introduction, use the literature to explain the background or rationale for conducting the research or project. Refer to the literature to demonstrate what has already been done to build your argument for why what you are writing is new, why it fills a gap, and why more work is needed in this area. In the discussion, use the literature to compare and contrast your findings with the findings of other studies on your topic. A thorough review of the literature empowers you to convince readers of your knowledge of the topic, to share what other researchers have shown to date, and to show how your study or project fits into the larger picture of the body of work on your research topic.

Avoiding Plagiarism

Plagiarism is taking someone else's words or ideas and presenting them as if they were your own, whether you do it knowingly or unknowingly. Whether plagiarism is unintentional or accidental—or blatant (i.e., knowingly and willfully committing plagiarism)—it is professional misconduct that can carry significant negative consequences such as revocation of degrees, dismissal from employment, hefty fines, and even incarceration. The vast majority of instances of plagiarism are unintentional, usually caused by not referencing things correctly in a manuscript's citations or quoting, paraphrasing, or summarizing someone's work without giving the original source proper credit. Findings from a 2014 study in the *Journal of Nursing Education* demonstrated that many postgraduate nursing and midwifery students "lack confidence in key referencing tasks" and that "incorrect referencing is rarely intentional and predominantly caused by skills deficit" (Greenwood et al., 2014, p. 447). In addition, the ease with which a copy-and-paste can be performed from a website or an electronic document is a potential pitfall contributing to unintentional plagiarism, particularly if the writer forgets to go back later and properly reference sources of information cut from various documents. The internet also blurs understanding of what is and is not considered "common knowledge"—information that anyone can look up in an online encyclopedia, for example, which does not need to be cited. Importantly, most peer-reviewed journals now employ automatic software that reviews all manuscripts for plagiarism before sending them out to reviewers; thus, regularly employing methods for avoiding plagiarism is essential. In your writing, pay close attention to when you are directly quoting a source versus when you are paraphrasing someone else's words versus when you are summarizing a large amount of information. Each of these requires a different approach to citing external references, and there are numerous ways through your writing style that you can clearly mark the boundaries between what needs to be cited versus what is your original work. Harris's *Using Sources Effectively: Strengthening Your Writing and Avoiding Plagiarism* is a practical and thorough resource for implementing these strategies and provides specific examples of how to mark the boundaries between your original thoughts and those that need to be cited (Harris, 2017). Also, you can check for plagiarism by running your manuscript through a software program.

Disseminating Findings at a Conference

Dissemination is the act of sharing your research study or project findings to obtain additional feedback from colleagues, stakeholders, or wider audience—either by oral (podium) or poster presentations at local, national, and international conferences. This is also a great opportunity to strategically network.

Choosing a Conference

If you are planning on writing an abstract for presentation, the first step is to target an appropriate conference. If you are a member of a professional organization, you will be on the email listserv it uses to share announcements about upcoming conferences and abstract submission opportunities (as well as calls for manuscripts). Even if you are not a member of an organization, it is sometimes possible to sign up for email listservs so you are notified of these opportunities. Most nationwide professional organizations have annual meetings, and some may also have smaller regional or chapter meetings to which you can submit abstracts. Choosing a conference requires steps similar to that of choosing an appropriate journal for a manuscript. Consider both large conferences that have broader, more inclusive foci as well as smaller, field-specific conferences to maximize your opportunities for dissemination. When you submit an abstract to a conference, you are typically given a choice to indicate whether you want it to be considered for an oral presentation, a poster presentation, or both. Choosing either or both may increase the likelihood that your abstract will be accepted since you are not limiting the options for selecting your abstract.

Another way to maximize dissemination opportunities is by turning conference presentations into articles for peer-reviewed journals. The study on changes in autism diagnosis rates is an example (Kulage et al., 2014). In May 2013, while the manuscript was being written, there was an opportunity to submit an abstract to the annual meeting of the International Society for Autism Research (INSAR). The manuscript was not complete; however, there was sufficient content, including results and conclusions, to submit an abstract. In September 2013, while the abstract was being reviewed by INSAR, the manuscript was completed and submitted it to the *Journal of Autism and Developmental Disorders*. That December the manuscript was accepted for publication. Less than a month later, the abstract was accepted for a poster presentation at the 2014 INSAR annual meeting. In February 2014, the article was published online ahead of print. In May, Kristine presented the poster at the INSAR conference, explaining to interested attendees that the peer-reviewed manuscript on this work was available online, and provided the complete reference on the printed poster. The article was printed in the July/August 2014 issue of the *Journal of Autism and Developmental Disorders*. This scenario demonstrates how a conference abstract and a manuscript can be developed in tandem, with the reviewing and acceptance processes going on simultaneously to maximize the impact of your work. Importantly, acceptance of an abstract for presentation does not preclude you from also writing up the work for a peer-reviewed publication unless the conference guidelines explicitly indicate that the work has not been presented elsewhere or submitted for publication.

Submitting an Abstract for Conference Presentation

For purposes of a manuscript, the *abstract* is a condensed and concentrated version of the full text and should represent the full scope of a study when read separately from the manuscript (Andrade, 2011). The goal of an abstract submitted to a conference for presentation is essentially the same, but importantly, this short (usually 200- to 300-word) document represents the full extent of the content that conference program committee members will consider when making recommendations on whether to accept an abstract for presentation. It should be well written, succinct, and accurately cover the main points of your study or project. Detailed information on writing effective abstracts for manuscripts and conferences is available in peer-reviewed journal articles (e.g., Andrade, 2011) and books (e.g., Oermann & Hays, 2018). More often than not, abstracts are structured and should include the following headings:

- Introduction or Background
- Aims
- Methods
- Results
- Conclusions

Other headings may be discussion and implications.

Some abstracts are unstructured and do not require headings; nevertheless, the same content would be provided. Be sure to follow the guidance provided by the journal or conference for which specific headings to include. Abstracts should also answer key questions about your study or project, such as:

- "What is already known about the topic?"
- "Why did you conduct the study or project?"
- "What did you do and how did you do it?"
- "What did you find and what do those findings mean?"

The scope of content you include in answering those questions will be limited by the number of words you are allotted, so as you revise, refine, and ultimately reduce the length of your abstract drafts, continually home in on the most important results for your readers. When you present your abstract via poster or orally, you will be able to expand on those elements. Because this is a stand-alone document, you want to avoid jargon and minimize the use of or eliminate acronyms. Finally, always avoid references and citations in abstracts; these can be included on a slide at the end of your PowerPoint presentation or printed on your poster.

Poster Presentations

A *poster* is a visual representation of a scholarly or research project or idea that is submitted to a conference for dissemination. As stated by Keely, nursing conferences use poster sessions "as a means to communicate innovative nursing practices and current research findings . . . in an interactive approach" (Keely, 2004, p. 182). In a poster you do not present every element of the study as you would in a manuscript. Within limited space, poster content shares a single message that is typically the most critical or influential finding of the project you conducted. The importance of delivering a single message should guide your poster development and revisions. In terms of career development and impacting the field, a poster also effectively advertises one element of your scholarly work.

Posters are a unique mechanism for sharing scholarly work because they prompt opportunities for conversation in a more personal way than oral presentations can achieve. A poster is a success if it gets your single message across to as many attendees as possible (Hess et al., 2014). Although you want to reach a large audience, most people will not stand in front of your poster and read every bullet point verbatim. The idea is that in a large room of 100 to 200 posters or more, you are trying to engage as many individuals walking down the aisles as possible to deliver your brief, single message, so take every opportunity to discuss your work one on one. Avoid the common pitfall of standing idly next to your poster watching attendees walk by, pause, glance over your work, and move on to the next poster. These are opportunities to actively engage peers in a discussion about your project and network with colleagues. Avoid the bad habit some presenters have adopted in which you secure your poster to the board and walk away. Make a commitment to stand by your poster for the entire session time, and take advantage of opportunities for scholarly exchange. A poster presentation can be a segue into a peer-reviewed article, so consider this for maximizing your project's exposure.

Designing the Poster

The best way to create a poster is to have it professionally printed as a single piece of paper, plastic, or cloth that maximizes the amount of space you have as dictated by the conference. A poster should follow the main headings that your abstract contained (i.e., introduction or background, aims, methods, results, and conclusions). You should refrain from reprinting your abstract on the poster (Hess et al., 2014; Mitrany, 2005). Any acknowledgments such as funding sources that supported the work should be listed. Because your abstract may be printed in a conference program or proceedings, it is important to present what you submitted. Prior to submitting your abstract for possible poster presentation, ensure that any future potential publication does not have any restriction against prepublication of your abstract. An exception is when a significant amount of time has elapsed since you submitted the abstract, and you have additional data or results now that may enhance your message. Because the content in the abstract will be shorter than what you can present a poster, you will want to expand on sections in your poster, primarily via graphics such as tables and figures. You can also include additional headings such as discussion, implications, future directions, references, and contact information. Use references sparingly; one strategy is that if your poster presents findings from a systematic literature review that included 30+ articles, include a handout of the full list of references for attendees, or just highlight a few key articles on the poster. A business card may be distributed as well instead of printing your phone number or email address on the poster.

Design your poster so that it is accessible to an audience both within and outside of your general area of expertise and poster topic. Content should not be provided only for specialists in your field. Do not omit essential contextual information assuming everyone will know why your topic is important and why they should care. Avoid jargon, and limit your use of field-specific acronyms. When you do use acronyms, make sure they are commonly recognized ones, and always spell them out at first use.

Posters can be designed using PowerPoint, but instead of creating multiple slides you will create your poster on a single slide that you will size according to conference guidelines. It is imperative that you follow conference guidelines for poster sizes: first, the maximum height and width, and second, whether posters should be horizontally or vertically oriented. All presenters are provided with a placard on which to append their posters, which should accommodate the dictated poster size. While you can use the entire space, you are not required to. To size your poster as a single slide, start with a blank PowerPoint file and customize your size as needed. Of note, PowerPoint has a maximum height and width allowable for a custom slide that will be a poster, which is 56 inches $\times$ 56 inches. If your poster needs to be a height or width that exceeds these maximum dimensions, you will need to take your size dimensions, in inches, and divide them in half, and use that for your custom settings for height and width. When you have it professionally printed, request that the poster be printed at *double* size. The key to ensuring the poster is printed appropriately is making sure your proportions remain the same for height and width to avoid stretching or pixilation when printing.

It is important to achieve proper balance in your poster through the placement of text and graphics to create something that is visually appealing. Balance occurs when images and text are reflected across a central axis, whether it is horizontal, vertical, or diagonal—this is known as the *axis of symmetry* (Hess et al., 2014). By using the axis of symmetry to guide your poster design, you ensure balance and avoid an asymmetrical poster (Hess et al., 2014).

Posters are a way to let graphics and images tell your story, so limit the amount of text used. Attendees will not want to stand and read your poster verbatim. An effective poster shows instead of tells (Kulage & Larson, 2016). When presenting your poster, you will engage in conversation, but your poster should show visitors what they need to know simply by looking at it. Thus, your take-home point should be emphasized, and tables, figures, graphs, and images should be used to summarize findings and illustrate main points whenever possible. In most cases, tables and figures are far more effective and efficient for presenting study results than narrative text. Make sure your graphics are of adequate size for viewers at a distance of several feet and are clean and simple enough to easily understand. A light-colored background with dark-colored letters for contrast is easier to read than light letters on a dark background. Use color to attract attention, organize similar items, or emphasize points, and stick to only a few colors, as more may overload and confuse your readers (Hess et al., 2014). Consider individuals with red/green color blindness and avoid using these colors if possible, particularly when they convey meaning. Finally, check if your institution's communication office has a standard or recommended layout, color scheme, or template for your use.

Avoid long lines of text in your poster by using phrases instead of full sentences. Bulleted or itemized lists are ideal. Use active voice in your phrasing, not passive, and pay attention to verb tense—if you are presenting on a completed study, use past tense throughout. Left justification of text is preferred over full justification for consistent word spacing and ease of reading. Headers and titles of graphics can, of course, be centered. It is commonly acknowledged that serif fonts, like Times New Roman, are easier to read and therefore recommended for posters. A good rule of thumb is that titles and major headings should be readable by someone standing 6 feet away from your poster, and the remaining material should be readable by someone standing 3 feet away. To test the font size of your poster before printing, Hess and colleagues suggest printing your poster on a standard size sheet of paper and then assessing how easily it can be read; if it is difficult to read, then your text will likely be too small for viewers when your large poster is printed (Hess et al., 2014).

Printing the Poster

There are several elements to consider when deciding how to print your poster: service, material, timing, shipping, travel convenience, and cost. There are basically two service options available for printing posters: brick-and-mortar store printing and online printing. You can bring an electronic copy of your poster on a flash drive to the store or access it on the store computer via email or a cloud service like DropBox.com or Microsoft's OneDrive. Staff will then print your poster, sometimes on the spot, but this option is usually limited to paper only with varying stock options (e.g., matte, glossy) that must remain rolled in a large tube for protection. If you are short on time, this may be your best option, and there are no shipping costs involved. Actual printing costs are largely determined by the paper stock and size of the poster.

For online printing, a Google search reveals numerous companies. Some brick-and-mortar stores also offer online printing options. These vendors allow you to upload your poster file to their website, after which they create a PDF proof of what it will look like printed, email it to you, and give you the opportunity to make edits before printing and shipping. Additionally, online stores usually offer multiple types of material including paper, plastic, cloth, and canvas.

When choosing your material, consider travel and costs—when using a brick-and-mortar store, printing on lightweight matte paper will be less expensive than glossy, heavyweight paper but will be less durable. If you are going to use the poster at multiple conferences, you may want to consider a more durable option and choose an online vendor that offers alternative material. Plastic and cloth posters can be easily folded for storage in a laptop case or briefcase for travel convenience instead of having a large tube as a plane carry-on. Foldable material will be more expensive but ultimately more feasible logistically. While all online vendors ship posters to their customers, some offer free shipping, and some may even ship your poster directly to the conference hotel. This can save travel woes and is helpful if you are short on time. Beware, though, that large conference hotels with business centers that offer the service of receiving your package may charge a fee ($20–$40) to hold your poster onsite until your arrival. If you are printing your poster at the last minute and require expedited printing, both brick-and-mortar and online stores will likely charge extra, so it is good practice to plan to have your poster printed a minimum of one week before the conference.

Making the Most of Your Poster Presentation Session

Even if the information you have displayed in your poster is clear, organized, easy to read, and visually appealing, your poster presentation during that one- to two-hour session will fall short if you fail to engage colleagues in discussion about your project. If someone pauses at your poster and begins to read or otherwise show interest, strike up a conversation. Ask them if they have any questions or if they would like you to summarize your poster, providing them with a verbal "tour" (Hess et al., 2014). Be prepared in advance having rehearsed your verbal overview. This exchange can help expedite further discussion about your project and its findings without leaving it to the viewer to stand and read your poster. A poster tour allows you to expand on details that may or may not be printed on your poster. Also, do not omit important contextual information in your tour by assuming everyone will know why your project is important or why they should care about your findings. And, as with poster design basics, avoid the use of verbal jargon in your tours.

A final suggestion to help your presentation continue to make an impact after the conference is the use of supplementary information. If possible, print small, one-page handouts of your posters on regular sized paper for your readers and, if applicable, reprints of published or in-press articles (as allowed by copyright law). These can be placed in an envelope and hung on the board with a thumbtack next to your poster. Also, freely distribute copies of your business card—poster presentations are ideal networking opportunities. Consider having a clipboard with pen and paper inviting comments from viewers or listing their names and email addresses should they want an electronic version of your poster. These information exchanges enable contact with colleagues at a later point in time, which could lead to future collaboration.

Oral (Podium) Presentations

There are two main elements to oral presentations at a conference: physical elements and accompanying slides. Although these are two distinct aspects, they go hand in hand because you are verbally walking your audience through your slides. Therefore, your physical presentation and content of your slides are equally important to ensure a high-quality presentation.

When you are speaking in front of a group of people, everyone can see your face and eyes and whether you're standing or sitting, making eye contact, or moving your hands or arms excessively. Therefore, it is important to be aware of your body language. First and foremost, always try to maintain eye contact with your audience. This is a good habit when you are describing a poster but even more important when giving an oral presentation. If you are behind a podium, stand up straight and maintain a stable, confident position facing the audience. There may be times you seem to be "tied" to the podium because of needing to see your slides on a laptop or using a microphone attached to the podium so you can be heard in a large room. Whenever possible, though, move around the room to engage your audience in your presentation. Part of that can be pointing out things on your slides, preferably with a laser pointer.

The most important tip for effective oral presentations is *not* to just read your slides to your audience, bullet by bullet, line by line. If that is all you are bringing to the face-to-face encounter with your audience, then your presentation will fall flat. There is no surer way to bore you audience than by reading your slides. Be engaging. Verbally expand on the brief, bulleted content you present on your slides, which essentially represents take-home points. Treat those bullets as cues to verify you are covering your main points. Speak loudly and clearly, adding variety to your speech and intonations, and avoid being robotic. Do not speak too quickly but in a measured yet natural pace. In fact, slowing down your speech is a good way to maintain control over your presentation.

It is often recommended that you "embrace the pause" when speaking to a crowd instead of filling those pauses with verbal "uhs" and "ums" that can irritate your audience and make you look unprepared. The "uhs" and "ums" can come rushing into the pauses of your speech when you are talking too quickly, when you have not fully rehearsed your presentation to gain a level of comfort with the content, when you have poorly planned or have no transitions between slides, or when you lack the confidence in what you are going to say next (McKay & McKay, 2012). Embracing the pause is a way to regain control over a presentation; let the silence of that pause allow you to regain your train of thought.

Make sure you are prepared for questions. Research in advance what questions audience members might ask during your presentation, and come prepared with answers. Formal and informal rehearsals are good for prompting potential questions, so take advantage of opportunities at your institution to rehearse your presentation before peers. However, someone may ask a question you may not be able to answer. In those cases, the right answer is: "Well, that's an excellent thought that I haven't considered, but in future work we will consider it." Better preparation and multiple rehearsals will not only reduce the "uhs" and "ums" in your speech but also improve the quality of your presentation.

The other essential element in oral presentations is the accompanying slides. But why use slides at all? First, they help promote effective communication with your audience, particularly when you have a limited amount of time to present. Slides help create a maximum impact in a minimal time and ensure a critical point is not omitted. Also, when you supplement what you are saying with a slide, you amplify your message by giving it verbally and visually. This combination accelerates the audience's ability to absorb information and improves their comprehension. However, keep in mind that PowerPoint is a slide manager, not a version of a word processing program, so keep text on slides to a minimum using bulleted phrases to highlight your major talking points, similar to the recommendations for poster presentations.

The number one pitfall to avoid in PowerPoint presentations is to have too many slides with too much content that cannot be amply covered in the time you are given. When you are giving an oral presentation at a conference, you will be given a specific time frame, typically somewhere between 10 minutes and 20 minutes, and when your time is up, you will be asked by a moderator to end the presentation so that all presentations remain on schedule. A feature in PowerPoint allows you to rehearse your presentation with a visible timing feature; if you know you have one minute per slide with 10 slides and 10 minutes total to speak, you can monitor your timing as you practice, making sure you remain within the limit.

The vast majority of the guidelines for recommended content and format for poster presentations are also applicable to PowerPoint slides. These include guidance on presenting a single message; presenting text in bulleted phrases instead of complete sentences; avoiding jargon and field-specific acronyms; using images when more effective than text; and considering color choices, font types, and overall consistency in formatting. In addition, the same guidance on rehearsing your presentation for posters applies to oral presentations. To highlight differences for slides, avoid distracting PowerPoint animation features, and use them only with a purpose so they do not take your audience's attention away from your take-home point. Also, anytime you can explain something clearly and succinctly in text in bulleted items with four or five words and a maximum of five bullets per slide, default to using text. A very busy graph or figure that attempts to show something that could be more easily explained in simple text can also distract your audience from your message. Text should be a minimum of 18-point font, with 24-point font ideal for larger headings. Finally, spot art can be used effectively to attract the attention of your audience and even add some humor to your presentation. And use spell check; just like manuscripts, it is amazing how often the spell check feature is neglected or simply forgotten.

Summary

Professional nurses have an ethical responsibility to disseminate the results of their studies at professional and scholarly forums locally, nationally, and internationally. Dissemination may be through publication, poster, and podium presentations. Dissemination is the process of sharing your study or project findings with colleagues and wider audiences to obtain additional feedback, publicize the results of your work, and advance nursing science, thus improving patient care outcomes.

Review Questions

1. Which of the following is (are) the common way(s) of disseminating study findings?

   A. Presenting at local, national, and international meetings of professional associations

   B. Publishing in a peer-reviewed journal

   C. Participating in poster presentations

   D. All of the above

   Answer: D. All of the above. Dissemination of study findings may occur through publication, poster, or podium presentations at scholarly forums or conferences that take place locally, nationally, and internationally.

2. Dissemination of research findings is an essential part of the research process because it adds to the body of knowledge in your area of expertise and contributes to improving patient care. True or False

   Answer: True. Dissemination is an intentionally developed approach to share knowledge and motivate others to change or improve patient care.

3. Dissemination is targeting study findings to specific journals, audiences, and stakeholders. True or False

Answer: True. Dissemination is intentional and must be targeted to specific audiences and stakeholders to effect change.

4. Which of the following best describes a good poster presentation?

 A. A good poster presentation must be visually attractive and capture the interest and attention of viewers.

 B. A good poster presentation must be readable, follow a logical sequence, and focus on key messages.

 C. A good poster presentation uses effective graphics, colors, and fonts.

 D. All of the above

Answer: D. A good poster presentation must be readable, clear, and to the point; visually attractive; and capture the interest of the readers.

5. Effective oral presentations mean:

 A. Presenter crams a 45-minute presentation into a 30-minute time slot to accommodate questions at the end of the session.

 B. Presenter is enthusiastic and engaging.

 C. Presenter reads slides line by line so as not to miss anything.

 D. All of the above

Answer: B. Presenter is enthusiastic and engaging. An effective oral presentation captures the audience's needs and interest and achieves the presenter's objectives. It is a dance between the presenter and the audience.

References

Andrade, C. (2011). How to write a good abstract for a scientific paper or conference presentation. *Indian Journal of Psychiatry, 53*(2), 172–175. http://www.indianjpsychiatry.org/article.asp?issn=0019-5545;year=2011;volume=53;issue=2;spage=172;epage=175;aulast=Andrade

Baerlocher, M. O., Newton, M., Gautam, T., Tomlinson, G., & Detsky, A. S. (2007). The meaning of author order in medical research. *Journal of Investigative Medicine, 55*(4), 174–180. http://dx.doi.org/10.2310/6650.2007.06044

Beall, J. (2012). Predatory publishers are corrupting open access. *Nature, 489*(7415), 179. https://www.nature.com/news/predatory-publishers-are-corrupting-open-access-1.11385

Cobey, K. D., Lalu, M. M., Skidmore, B., Ahmadzai, N., Grudniewicz, A., & Moher, D. (2018). What is a predatory journal? A scoping review. *F1000Research, 7*, 1001. https://f1000research.com/articles/7-1001

Garfield, E. (2006). The history and meaning of the journal impact factor. *JAMA, 295*(1), 90–93. https://jamanetwork.com/journals/jama/article-abstract/202114

Greenwood, M., Walkem, K., Smith, L. M., Shearer, T., & Stirling, C. (2014). Post-graduate nursing student knowledge, attitudes, skills, and confidence in appropriately referencing academic work. *Journal of Nursing Education, 53*(8), 447–452.

Harris, R. A. (2017). *Using sources effectively: Strengthening your writing and avoiding plagiarism* (5th ed.). Routledge.

Hess, G., Tosney, K., & Liegel, L. (2014). *Creating effective poster presentations.* http://www.ncsu.edu/project/posters

International Committee of Medical Journal Editors. (2010). Uniform requirements for manuscripts submitted to biomedical journals: Writing and editing for biomedical publication. *Journal of Pharmacology & Pharmacotherapeutics, 1*(1), 42–58.

Keely, B. R. (2004). Planning and creating effective scientific posters. *Journal of Continuing Education in Nursing, 35*(4), 182–185.

Kulage, K. M., & Larson, E. L. (2016). Implementation and outcomes of a faculty-based, peer review manuscript writing workshop. *Journal of Professional Nursing, 32*(4), 262–270.

Kulage, K. M., Smaldone, A. M., & Cohn, E. G. (2014). How will DSM-5 affect autism diagnosis? A systematic literature review and meta-analysis. *Journal of Autism and Developmental Disorders, 44*(8), 1918–1932. https://link.springer.com/article/10.1007/s10803-014-2065-2

McKay, G., & McKay, K. (2012). Becoming well-spoken: How to minimize your uh's and um's. *The art of manliness.* https://www.artofmanliness.com/articles/becoming-well-spoken-how-to-minimize-your-uhs-and-ums/

Mitrany, D. (2005). Creating effective poster presentations: The editor's role. *Science Editor, 28*(4), 114–116.

Morton, P. G. (2013). Publishing in professional journals, part I: Getting started. *AACN Advanced Critical Care, 24*(2), 162–168.

Oermann, M. H., & Hays, J. C. (2018). *Writing for publication in nursing* (4th ed.). Springer Publishing Company.

PEACE MODEL

P | **PROBLEM IDENTIFICATION**
Formulate the clinical question (**PICO**):
- **P** | Patient Population
- **I** | Intervention
- **C** | Comparison of Intervention
- **O** | Outcome

E | **EVIDENCE REVIEW**
Review evidence relevant to your clinical question by searching databases.

A | **APPRAISE EVIDENCE**
Appraise the evidence that appears highest in the hierarchy of scientific evidence for its quality and applicability to practice.

C | **CHANGE PRACTICE OR CONDUCT RESEARCH**
If evidence is sufficient, embark on improvement project to address practice change.
If evidence is insufficient to warrant practice change, conduct research.

E | **EVALUATE AND DISSEMINATE FINDINGS**
Evaluate the impact of the implemented practice change and research results.
Disseminate findings through publication, oral, and poster presentations.

9

RESOURCES

–Laarni C. Florencio, MSN, RN, CNL | Warly Remegio, DNP, MS, RN-BC, CCRN-CSC

KEYWORDS | PHRASES
evidence-based practice, practice focused inquiry,
culture of inquiry, EBP and research resources, clinical practice guidelines,
professional practice model, nursing strategic plan, PEACE model, EBP models,
professional governance councils, nurse scientists, critical appraisal tools

CHAPTER OBJECTIVES

After studying this chapter, learners will be able to:

1. Describe their organization's EBP model.
2. Enumerate resources needed when conducting EBP projects.
3. Identify the organizational infrastructure involved in their EBP process.

Introduction

Clinicians embarking on an evidence-based practice (EBP) project are often faced with where and how to tackle the breadth of evidence relevant to their work. Learning how to navigate your organization's research infrastructure helps with knowledge translation. It starts with the integration of the EBP process in your employee orientation. The introduction to the EBP model your organization adheres to determines the foundational path to ignite your own practice-focused inquiry. At NewYork-Presbyterian (NYP), we are committed to providing access to high-quality scientific evidence and fostering an environment suitable for research and EBP implementation.

Melnyk and Fineout-Overholt (2019) have cited how EBP is effective in improving patient experiences. Its implementation has been documented to achieve better patient outcomes. However, multiple factors also affect the successful translation of these evidences to practice. It is advisable to adhere to effective knowledge management skills to be able to adequately process and sift through resources effectively.

The figures discussed in this chapter illustrate the resources clinicians can use for their EBP projects at NYP (see Figure 9.1). Various resources have been outlined in this chapter to provide guidance and information to any of our staff embarking on improving processes using EBP at the point of care.

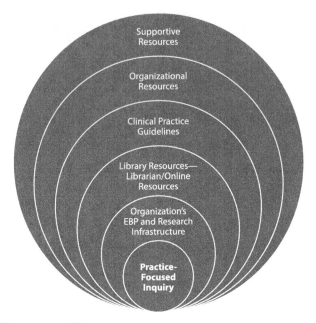

Figure 9.1 | EBP resources at NYP.

Organizational Research Infrastructure and Foundation

A culture of inquiry is developed and further enhanced by an organization's commitment and effort to provide an environment conducive for knowledge discovery and best practice implementation. It begins with laying the foundation of fundamental knowledge related to EBP and research.

A look at your organization's professional practice model (see Figure 9.2), EBP model, and strategic plan (see Figure 9.3) will serve as a guide to help steer your EBP project. These will serve as your north star in determining areas of relevant study and opportunities for practice improvement. Knowing the fundamental research infrastructure of your organization will be key in the management and translation of evidence as you go along. It is essential to know this information as baseline tools to your success.

NYP Professional Practice Model

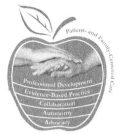

- **Advocacy:** Empower patients, families, communities, and colleagues to ensure culturally competent and compassionate care

- **Autonomy:** Foster self-directed practice through critical thinking and accountability

- **Collaboration:** Promote interprofessional communication and coordination of patient/family-centered care

- **Evidence-Based Practice:** Integrate clinical expertise, scientific findings, and patient preference to improve outcomes

- **Professional Development:** Commit to personal, clinical, and scholarly growth to optimize the patient experience

NewYork-Presbyterian
The image represents the Big Apple, with the hands depicting the warm relationship between nurses and patients and families. This relationship is built on the five essential elements of nursing practice, unified by one purpose: patient and family-centered care.

Figure 9.2 | NYP professional practice model.

NewYork-Presbyterian
Department of Nursing

Nursing Strategic Plan 2018–2021

Themes/Areas of Focus	Professional Practice Model	What We Want to Accomplish
Professional Development and Education (PDE)	Professional Development	-Standardize NYP Nursing Professional Development structures and functions across the enterprise to promote a culture of continuous learning and interprofessional collaboration. -Implement the use of innovative technology, such as simulation and other platforms to enhance engagement and optimize learning. -Leverage the resources at NYP to implement globally recognized educational opportunities and leadership development at all levels of practice.
Quality and Safety (QS)	Evidence-Based Practice	-Standardize and integrate Nursing Quality Safety program across enterprise. -Progress toward High Reliability Nursing Organization. -Improve nursing engagement in quality and safety activities.
Advancing Care (AC)	Professional Development/ Evidence-Based Practice/ Collaboration/Autonomy/ Advocacy	-Evaluate professional governance and professional practice model. -Improve infrastructure to share and integrate best practices. -Expand research fellowship program at all campuses.
Operational Excellence (OE)	Collaboration/Advocacy	-Foster a culture of ownership of individual role on organization's financial goals. -Create Finance Councils across NewYork-Presbyterian. -Leverage financial technology platforms. -Explore alternate staffing models. -Lead the organization in financial stewardship.
Technology Innovation (TI)	Evidence-Based Practice/ Collaboration/ Autonomy	-Develop nursing teams to participate in Electronic Health Record project. -Build on mobility platform to create nursing efficiencies. -Leverage artificial intelligence and telenursing. -Standardize technology across NewYork-Presbyterian. -Empower nurses to use technology to drive efficiency and safety.
Nursing Engagement (NX)	Collaboration/ Autonomy/ Advocacy	-Improve culture of respect and workforce diversity. -Strive toward zero harm. -Improve quality and modes of communication within and between campuses. -Promote a culture of engagement, accountability, and collaboration. -Recruit and retain top talent.
Patient-Family Experience (PFX)	Collaboration/ Autonomy/ Advocacy	-Improve quality and modes of communication. -Improve HCAHPS responsiveness scores. -Improve interprofessional collaboration and care coordination.

Figure 9.3 | NYP's nursing strategic plan.

Flowchart of Steps: Conducting Nursing Evidence-Based Practice and Research at NewYork-Presbyterian

The clinical nurse is essential to building a culture of inquiry to advance nursing science and improve patient care.

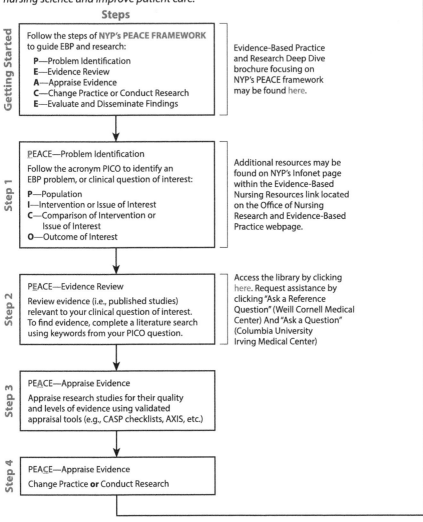

Steps

Getting Started

Follow the steps of **NYP's PEACE FRAMEWORK** to guide EBP and research:

P—Problem Identification
E—Evidence Review
A—Appraise Evidence
C—Change Practice or Conduct Research
E—Evaluate and Disseminate Findings

Evidence-Based Practice and Research Deep Dive brochure focusing on NYP's PEACE framework may be found here.

Step 1

P**E**ACE—Problem Identification

Follow the acronym PICO to identify an EBP problem, or clinical question of interest:

P—Population
I—Intervention or Issue of Interest
C—Comparison of Intervention or Issue of Interest
O—Outcome of Interest

Additional resources may be found on NYP's Infonet page within the Evidence-Based Nursing Resources link located on the Office of Nursing Research and Evidence-Based Practice webpage.

Step 2

PE**A**CE—Evidence Review

Review evidence (i.e., published studies) relevant to your clinical question of interest. To find evidence, complete a literature search using keywords from your PICO question.

Access the library by clicking here. Request assistance by clicking "Ask a Reference Question" (Weill Cornell Medical Center) And "Ask a Question" (Columbia University Irving Medical Center)

Step 3

PEA**C**E—Appraise Evidence

Appraise research studies for their quality and levels of evidence using validated appraisal tools (e.g., CASP checklists, AXIS, etc.)

Step 4

PEAC**E**—Appraise Evidence

Change Practice **or** Conduct Research

Figure 9.4 | PEACE model flowchart for EBP and research.

Step 4A—Change Practice

PEACE—Change Practice

If **evidence is sufficient**, recommend a change in practice to the Nursing Practice Council and to the Director of Nursing Research and Innovation. Information on the Office of Professional Nursing Practice may be found here.

Professional Governance Resource Handbook may be found here.

Contact information for the Director of Nursing Research and Innovation may be found here.

Step 4B—Conduct Research

PEACE—Conduct Research

If **evidence is sufficient**, conduct research. Prepare and submit your nursing research proposal to the Director of Nursing Research and Innovation and to the chair of your campus's Nursing EBP and Research Council. For contact information, click here. Present your proposal to members of your campus Nursing Research and EBP Council. The Director of Nursing Research and Innovation will share the recommended research proposals with the Vice President of Nursing. Council chair(s) and the Director of Nursing Research and Innovation will facilitate additional approvals, as needed.

Work with the Campus Nurse Researcher to submit your institutional review board (IRB) protocol. Prior to submitting your IRB protocol, you must complete the required human subjects research training modules. East campuses (Lower Manhattan, Weill Cornell and Westchester), access CITI Program through WRG. You need to create an account and register; click here. Choose Weill Cornell Medical College as your affiliation and complete the (1) Human Subjects Research in Biomedical Research and (2) Good Clinical Practice modules. Then follow additional Weill Research Gateway (WRG) requirements. West campuses (Columbia, Allen, MSCH, Lawrence, and Hudson Valley), call 4-HELP for UNI and complete HIPAA, conflict of interests form, and Human Subjects Protection (HSP) training. For HSP training, select Columbia University as your affiliation. NYP Queens and NYP Brooklyn Methodist have their own IRB and may access their account through CITI Program.

The study may only begin after IRB approval.

Step 5

PEACE—Evaluate and Disseminate Findings

Evaluate impact of the implemented practice change or research specified in the PICO question. When evaluating impact of practice change, you may apply the Performance Improvement/Quality Improvement Process or Squire Guidelines.

Step 6

Present findings at NYP sponsored forums **and** prepare findings for publication. Be sure to inform the Director of Nursing Research and Innovation of the publications and presentations that result from your EBP and research projects!

The PEACE model flowchart for EBP and research (Figure 9.4) provides step-by-step guidelines in utilizing the PEACE model and the resources that are available for nurses. This important tool will assist nurses to stay on course and on point in building a culture of inquiry.

The Library

Knowledge creation starts with a robust and abundant resource of information. Searching for relevant knowledge sources is an essential component of the EBP process. There is no better source than the library (see Figure 9.5). It houses your first-generation knowledge (primary studies such as randomized trials and interrupted time series), second-generation knowledge (such as systematic reviews), and third-generation knowledge (such as tools, decision aides, and educational models; Strauss et al., 2009).

LIBRARY RESOURCES

For treatment questions: Systematic reviews of randomized controlled trials
For meaning questions: Meta-syntheses of qualitative studies
For prognosis or prediction questions: Syntheses of cohort case-control studies
For diagnosis questions: Syntheses of randomized control trials or cohort studies
For etiology questions: Syntheses of cohort or case-control studies

ESP Resources and Databases:

Helene Fund Health Trust National Institute for EBP in Nursing and Healthcare at the Ohio State University College of Nursing

Joanna Briggs Institute (JBI) Evidence Based Practice Database

The Sarah Cole Hirsch Institute for Evidence Based Practice at Case Western Reserve School of Nursing

The Johns Hopkins Nursing Center for Evidence Based Practice at Johns Hopkins University

Other Pertinent Databases:

Health-related research: MEDLINE, EMBASE, The Cochrane Central Register of Controlled Trials
Subject-specific databases: Cumulative Index of Nursing and Allied Health (CINAHL)
Geographical databases: Latin American Caribbean Health Sciences Literature (LILACS)

Figure 9.5 | Library resources.

An even better resource is librarians. Their expertise can help locate and select studies and trial registers and search through a broad screen of citations and full-text articles. They can also help navigate online resources. Most important is that librarians can help determine the best relevant resources available to you based on your identified problem.

The expertise of the librarian can help with database searches electronically, whether bibliographic, geographical, or subject-specific. They can assist you in selecting, navigating, and reviewing various databases such as Medline, EMBASE, Cochrane Central Register of Controlled Trials, Cumulative Index of Nursing and Allied Health, and Latin American Caribbean Health Sciences Literature (Strauss, et al., 2009). The components of your PICO question determine the source for relevant studies. This is why it is imperative to consult the librarian to effectively traverse and manage comprehensive databases for your study. Figure 9.6 illustrates the different resources that may be helpful depending on which stage of the PEACE model you are working on.

PEACE Model	Organizational Research Infrastructure	Library	Organizational Resources	Clinical Practice Guidelines	Supportive Resources
(P)roblem identification Practice-focused inquiry/PICO question	x	x	x	x	
(E)vidence review		x			
(A)ppraise evidence			x		x
(C)onduct research/ change practice			x	x	x
(E)valuate practice change			x	x	x

Figure 9.6 | Appropriate resources for PEACE model.

Practice-based inquiry is an effective research strategy that generates accurate findings about the quality of interventions implemented in real time in current situations. To use it effectively, it necessitates the rigor that ensures the accuracy, credibility, and legitimacy of the findings and resources. It is about asking great, thoughtful questions based on what is currently happening and on what relevant information is on hand. Knowing the resources available and understanding the interplay and connectivity of the resources fosters the organized management of information directed to lead to meaningful and well-thought-out PICO questions and a palpable culture of inquiry.

Clinical Practice Guidelines

Evidence-based *clinical practice guidelines* are systematically developed statements that assist clinicians and patients to make appropriate healthcare decisions regarding specific clinical circumstances (IOM, 1990). They are knowledge tools that aim to assist in healthcare decision-making. Clinical practice guidelines facilitate high-quality practice supported by evidence. They allow for appropriate resource allocation and advance research by identifying research gaps and areas in which additional research can be done.

They are suitable EBP resources primarily because they define the role of specific diagnostic and treatment modalities in the diagnosis and management of patients. They contain recommendations that are based on evidence taken from rigorous systematic reviews and synthesis of published health literatures. They are not set in stone but are usually followed with the intent to manage care effectively and appropriately.

An understanding of these guidelines will aid clinicians in problem identification, conducting their research, facilitating change in practice, and evaluating their interventions. A list of clinical practice guidelines can be found at https://nccih.nih.gov/health/providers/clinicalpractice.htm.

Organizational Resources

The commitment and support of an organization to provide evidence-based care stems from the adequate provision of fundamental and foundational resources to promote the growing culture of inquiry and best practice implementation. Critical to any clinician's success engaging in any EBP, process improvement, research, or quality work would be the accessibility to these resources. Following are additional collaborative and supportive resources, unique to organizations that promote an environment conducive for best practice inquiry and implementation.

Professional Governance Councils (EBP and Research, Education Staff Councils)

The EBP and research committee is part of the professional governance structure that aims to support and facilitate the advancement of research and innovation among nurses throughout an organization. Its ultimate goal is to expand nurses' knowledge, skills, and abilities to critically appraise scientific articles for quality and evaluate studies for clinical relevance in improving patient care outcomes and the general delivery of care.

The committee is an essential resource for EBP and research because it provides nurses a platform to discuss how to elevate their practice at the clinical setting. Committee members are composed of nurse leaders, nurse educators, advanced practice nurses, clinical nurse scientists, nursing faculty from affiliated schools and colleges of nursing, and clinical nurses from various practice areas.

Committee members partake in supporting the ethical conduct of research, ensuring the accurate record of nursing-led research initiatives; developing mechanisms for increasing nursing research visibility within the institution as well as regionally, nationally, and internationally; and working with other professional governance venues including unit councils and other organizational committees (such as quality and safety, and practice) in facilitating EBP and research.

The monthly committee meetings serve as a forum for members to discuss operational barriers and opportunities in promoting a culture of inquiry. The committee serves as the primary gatekeeper for potential EBP, quality improvement (QI), and research projects in the organization. Consultation and feedback are provided to nurses who present their PICO questions or research abstracts during the meeting. The committee's clinical researcher and other experts provide guidance on the design, interventions, and research protocols and outcome measures of the project. This engaging learning activity expands the participants' knowledge on research and EBP as they gain mentorship and guidance based on the discussions and feedback given by subject matter experts.

Journal Clubs

Healthcare organizations are utilizing journal clubs in furthering nurses' appreciation and engagement in research and EBP. They are conducted at the unit, service line, or organizational level. Journal clubs are often established to discuss scientific articles and their relevance to current nursing practice. Nursing journal clubs aim to develop nurses' ability to appraise articles, enhance their knowledge on research terms and methodologies, and hone their skills in interpreting research findings and in evaluating the relevance of the studies to their current specialty. Nurses' continuous involvement with these activities further stirs their interests in embracing clinical scientific inquiry. Journal clubs significantly facilitate the integration of EBP in the clinical setting.

Subject Matter Experts (SMEs) in EBP and Research

Subject matter experts are highly trained individuals specializing in EBP and research. They have a high level of understanding regarding processes of EBP, performance improvement, and research. They serve as a valuable resource for nurses in various stages of the EBP/research process. Identified SMEs within the organization include nurse scientists, nursing professional development specialists, nurse leaders, quality and patient safety coordinators or officers, clinical nurse specialists, and expert clinicians.

Nurse Scientists

Nurse scientists are PhD-prepared nurses who lend support to clinical nurses engaged in EBP and research projects. At NYP, nurse scientists lead monthly nursing grand rounds on EBP and research, conduct EBP workshops, and facilitate research and EBP symposia. They provide one-on-one mentorship and support to nurses interested in pursuing EBP, QI, or research projects within and outside the EBP fellowship programs. Nurse scientists support the advancement of research in both the academic and the clinical settings to reconcile the gaps in practice between both settings.

Volunteer Members of the Academic Partners Program

The development of the Academic Partners Program (APP) enriches the resources of EBP and research in the organization. Similar to the goals of having dually appointed nursing scientists, the APP's goal is to expand the resources for EBP and research and to further support the collaborative partnerships of healthcare and academia in the area of research toward improving nursing education and healthcare delivery. At NYP, the volunteer faculty from affiliate colleges and universities serve as the academic liaison, participating in the hospital's EBP/research committee meetings. As core members of the committee, they lend their academic and research expertise to the nurses. They introduce potential healthcare research initiatives that may have some impact on nursing and healthcare delivery.

Nursing Professional Development Specialists

Nursing professional development (NPD) specialists play an integral role as a resource for EBP and research. NPD specialists act as champions of scientific inquiry, generating new knowledge and integrating best available evidence into practice (Harper & Maloney, 2016). The NPD specialists' clinical expertise, strong background in EBP and research, and mentoring abilities make them a suitable resource for EBP in the organization.

At NYP, NPD specialists have integrated EBP in their orientation curriculum and in their general onboarding competency, utilizing the Quality and Safety Education for Nurses framework. The NPD specialist teaches the NYP EBP PEACE model in orientation and emphasizes how EBP is weaved into NYP's professional practice model and in the department of nursing's strategic plan. This structure leverages the nurses' clinical practice as they embrace EBP from the beginning of their career in the organization.

Additionally, NPD specialists have significant roles in the clinical nurses' day-to-day practice. They serve as active resources in reconciling practice gaps in the clinical setting. They are responsible for maintaining the competencies of clinical nurses by providing ongoing education and professional development opportunities. They provide mentoring to clinical nurses who are aspiring to be part of the clinical ladder program. This program entails the development and implementation of an EBP, QI, or research project. NPD provides open consultation hours and workshops to clinical nurses to guide them in their pursuit of the clinical ladder program.

NPD and the office of research and innovation work collaboratively in implementing professional development initiatives to build and enhance the competencies of nurses in EBP, QI, and research. Examples of these education initiatives include nursing grand rounds, clinical ladder workshops, EBP deep dive, EBP and research symposia, and writing publications. These programs have been successfully implemented at NYP Hospital and across the enterprise.

Patient Safety, Risk, and Quality Officers

The members of quality and patient safety, work health and safety, and infection prevention are valuable resources for EBP, QI, and research. These individuals promote action through implementation of proven methods that can be EBP, research, or QI. They have tremendous expertise in trending and interpreting data and in collaborating with various stakeholders toward implementing change. Nurses can utilize them as resources because they can identify opportunities and practice gaps or evaluate the effectiveness of their interventions.

Advanced Practice Registered Nurses

Advanced practice registered nurses (APRNs) are a valuable resource for EBP, QI, and research. They provide primary, acute, and specialty healthcare across the life span through assessment, diagnosis, and treatment of illnesses and injuries utilizing evidence-based medicine. They meticulously examine the application of current treatment protocols and clinical practice guidelines to ensure the provision of safe and quality care. APRNs include nurse practitioners, clinical nurse specialists, nurse anesthetists, and nurse midwives. All play an integral role in advancing the future of healthcare.

Nurse Managers/Nurse Leaders

Nurse leaders play a pivotal role in influencing nursing practice and in changing an organizational or unit culture. Nurse leaders' expertise in collaboration and system thinking, resource management, and benchmarking is beneficial in facilitating the success of implementing EBP, QI, and research. Additionally, they serve as mentors as they continue to guide and grow the abilities of their subordinates through performance evaluation.

Research and EBP Fellowship Programs

Healthcare organizations recognize the tremendous need for EBP in guiding healthcare delivery. Regulatory and accrediting bodies and consumers underscore the importance of infusing EBP at the point of care to improve patient care outcome. This poses a daunting challenge to most healthcare leaders as they are faced with scarce resources not only in educating nurses but also in hardwiring this concept in the organizational culture. Healthcare organizations recognize the need for EBP mentors, who are effective in educating and supporting clinical nurses in implementing evidence-based care.

At NYP, an innovative program, the LINK project, was developed to address the lack of education and lack of EBP resources within the organization. This clinical-academic partnership initiative created a formal command and control structure bringing together existing academic resources, including the PhD-prepared nurse researcher, a biostatistician, and the development of a formal research consultation request process (Cato et al., 2019). This further improved the consolidation of ongoing and growing collaborations between clinical and academic settings, leveraging the statistical, research design, and research project management expertise available at the school of nursing to support the clinical nurses in the successful completion of the research project from conceptualization to dissemination (Cato et al., 2019). This program received consistently positive feedback from clinical nurses, nurse leaders, nurse researchers, and other stakeholders of the organization. This robust and streamlined resource initiative, in addition to the aforementioned resources, strengthened the collaborative partnership of the university and the school toward advancing EBP and research, which are the markers for excellence.

Furthermore, NYP implemented the EBP fellowship program on all its campuses to further advance EBP and research throughout the organization. This avenue provides more opportunities for collaborative training, mentoring, and support to direct care RNs who can take back the new knowledge, skills, and abilities to the bedside care environment. The structure of EBP fellowship programs is designed to allow the fellows to develop a project that is meaningful to the organization. Each fellow has access to one or more mentors and the EBP faculty in the organization.

Supportive Resources

Supportive resources complement existing EBP resources to further aggrandize the current innovative EBP structures in fostering a culture of inquiry among clinical nurses. These resources contribute largely to the development of a relevant PICO question and the selection of the most appropriate information, and they add rigor to the evidence and validate effectiveness of best practices and outcomes. They are tools that help with appraisal, add value to the evidence or outcomes of the interventions implemented, and develop further one's skill in carrying out the EBP process.

EBP Workshops and Training

EBP workshops and training further enhance one's skill set in doing EBP projects. They also promote familiarity with the process and widen one's ability to manage information and knowledge translation. Organizations such as NYP fully understand that providing these courses contribute to the growth and expertise of any clinical nurse interested in EBP. Courses like those listed in Figure 9.7 contribute to the organization's commitment to empower their nurses in elevating their practice.

Nursing Professional Development Programs and Innovation & Research	Topics

Nursing grand rounds: PEACE model
 	
• A 1-hour program series designed to introduce to the participants the different elements of the PEACE model
	• Overview of EBP and the PEACE model
	• Problem identification
	  • What constitutes a problem
	  • Formulating a PICO question
	• Evidence review
	  • Different levels of evidence
	  • Where to look for sources of evidence (i.e., library services, journal articles, professional organizations' websites, clinical practice guidelines)
	  • How to do basic literature search
	• Appraising the evidence
	  • Evidence appraisal templates
	  • Synthesis and recommendation tools
	• Change of practice/change of policy
	  • Synthesis of the evidence
	  • Fit, feasibility, and appropriateness of practice change
	• Evaluation & dissemination of findings
	  • Evaluation of practice changes/findings

Clinical ladder workshop • A 4.5-hour program designed to assist the participants in their successful application to the clinical ladder program	• Overview of the clinical ladder program (goals and objectives, structures, and process) • The differences between EBP, QI, and research, including some exemplars • Resources, exemplars, strategies, and tools (REST) for implementing EBP, QI, and research • Project management

EBP deep dive	• Problem identification
A 7.0-hour program designed to assist the participants in developing an EBP project or research	• Evidence review terminology
	• Appraise the evidence
	• Change practice
	• Conduct research
	• Difference between EBP, research, and QI
	• Quantitative research, qualitative research, and mixed methods
	• Ethics in research
	• Data analysis/validity/reliability
	• CITI training
	• Project management
	• Evaluation and dissemination of findings
	• Poster presentations
	• Squire guidelines
	• Journal club
	• Publications
	• Resources for EBP and research

Figure 9.7 | EBP courses at NYP.

Critical Appraisal Tools

Critical appraisal tools help in the appraisal of various types of evidence. They aid in assessing the relevance, trustworthiness, and accuracy of research results. These tools allow one to systematically evaluate clarity in the research question, whether the researchers used valid methods to address the research question, whether the results are important to the study, and whether the outcomes are applicable to practice. One can choose from various appraisal tools. The most common is the Critical Appraisal Skills Programme. This tool has 10 to 12 questions pertaining to validity, outcomes, and relevance. The tool assesses systematic reviews, randomized controlled trials, qualitative research, economic evaluation studies, cohort studies, case control studies, and diagnostic test studies.

Quality Outcomes

Quality indicator systems such as the Agency for Healthcare Research and Quality (AHRQ) National Healthcare Quality Report, National Quality Forum (NQF), and National Database of Nursing Quality Indicators (NDNQI) provide insightful evidence of quality care outcomes over a period of time. These reports are significant in evaluating the effectiveness and sustainability of evidence implementation. The information they provide allows us to look at the impact of innovations to practice and overall outcomes. They provide vital opportunities for improvement and comparison of results with national benchmarks:

- **AHRQ National Healthcare Quality Report** is an annual report that monitors the nation's state of healthcare quality. It extensively measures care effectiveness and efficiency, timeliness of care, patient safety, and patient-centered care. The report outlines opportunities for improvement in preventive care, management of chronic diseases, and other patient safety outcomes.

- **National Quality Forum (NQF)** came up with nursing-sensitive measures, consensus-based nursing standards for inpatient care. They measure processes and outcomes that are influenced by and provided by nursing. This report highlights the contributions of nursing to patient-centered outcomes, nursing-centered interventions, and system-centered measures. By measuring skill mix, nurse staffing hours, prevalence of pressure ulcers and patient falls, smoking cessation counseling, and nursing care hours per patient day, NQF was able to establish the relationship among patient care outcomes, nursing productivity, and healthcare costs.

- **NDNQI reports on factors influencing nursing care** is a nursing database that provides quarterly and annual reports highlighting the structure, process, and outcome indicators to evaluate nursing care at the unit level. It depicts how nursing performance impacts patient outcomes. It allows healthcare organizations to identify opportunities for improvement at the unit level. Its primary goal is to assist the clinical nurse in improving patient safety and QI efforts by providing national comparative data that are research-based (NDNQI, 2010).

Point-of-Care Resources

Clinical nurses can utilize different resources at the point of care. These resources include the use of case studies, anecdotal reports, incident/patient safety reports, the unit data for clinical quality indicators, results of patient rounding, and patient experience (such as Hospital Consumer Assessment of Healthcare Providers and Systems scores). Point-of-care resources are helpful in pinpointing situations clearly unique to a specific department, patient population, or practice. These captured circumstances may not be experienced in general healthcare circumstances. These data will guide nurses in identifying practice gaps for further QI initiatives and evidence-based projects or research.

Every organization has an array of resources for nurses to do an EBP project. Healthcare organizations such as NYP realize the importance of best practice in providing the most effective care that is available. It can be achieved by fostering a culture of inquiry, an integration of research evidence into practice, and a collaborative healthcare environment committed to best practice implementation and evaluation.

Summary

There are abundant resources available in every organization supportive of the EBP process. In addition to infrastructural resources, interprofessional collaboration, professional governance, and academic partnerships are essential forms of resources supportive of the successful development and sustainability of a culture of inquiry.

Identified EBP resources fully serve their purpose when they are easily accessible, readily available, and deemed appropriate by those that need them the most. Healthcare organizations such as NYP recognize the value of these resources and have continually and consistently provided innovative ways to support the enculturation of best practices.

Ultimately, resources for EBP can be cultivated in any organization that is committed to fostering a culture of inquiry (Spiva et al., 2017). The EBP resources covered in this chapter facilitate the seamless integration of research evidence into practice toward improving care delivery and patient care outcomes. Therefore, organizations must continue to embrace a collaborative healthcare environment to sustain and expand these resources.

Review Questions

1. What is your organization's EBP model?

   Answer: There are various EBP models to choose from. NYP specifically uses the PEACE EBP model. The model is extensively discussed in this book. Your organization's EBP model is usually introduced to you at the beginning of your orientation. The culture, practice, and implementation of EBP and research in your organization are sustained by several programs and resources, which are also discussed at length in this chapter of the book.

2. What are your organization's EBP resources for a successful implementation of an EBP project?

   Answer: A variety of tools and resources are usually available to any organization to help with the successful implementation of any EBP project. There is a myriad of organizational resources such as professional governance councils and journal clubs that help disseminate information regarding EBP. The library is also a prime resource for peer-reviewed articles and well-established publications supporting best practice and evidence-based studies. There are several other resources mentioned in this chapter for everyone's reference and use.

3. What is the role of your professional governance councils in EBP or research?

   Answer: The professional governance councils support and facilitate the advancement of research and innovation among nurses throughout an organization. They help with teaching nurses how to critically appraise scientific articles for clinical relevance. They are an essential resource to the staff in terms of EBP and research education, knowledge translation, best practice dissemination, and translation of EBP to practice.

4. How are EBP and research promoted and sustained in your organization?

   Answer: A strong EBP and research core structure and foundation is key in building and maintaining the culture of inquiry in your organization. Once it is ingrained in your healthcare system, it becomes part of everyone's practice in your organization. Establishing key strategies such as nursing professional development and clinical ladder programs enhances and sustains the translation of EBP knowledge to practice consistently.

5. What is the organizational infrastructure involved in your EBP process?

   Answer: It starts with the foundation of fundamental knowledge related to EBP and research. Your organization's professional practice model, EBP model, and strategic plan serve as guides for practice improvement. Knowing the fundamental research infrastructure of your organization will be key in the translation of evidence as you improve and render high-quality EBP. It is essential to know this information as baseline tools to your success.

References

Cato, K. D., Sun, C., Carter, E., Liu, J., Rivera, R., & Larson, E. (2019). Linking to improve nursing care and knowledge. Evaluation of an initiative to provide research support to clinical nurses. *Journal of Nursing Administration, 49*(1), 48–54.

Harper, M. G., & Maloney, P. (Eds.). (2016). Nursing professional development: Scope and standards of practice (3rd ed.). Chicago, IL: ANPD.

Institute of Medicine (IOM). (1990). Clinical practice guidelines: Directions for a new program. Washington DC: National Academy Press.

National Database of Nursing Quality Indicators (NDNQI). (2010). NDNQI: Transforming data into quality care.

Melnyk, B., & Fineout-Overholt, E. (2019). *Evidence-based practice in nursing and healthcare* (4th ed.). Wolters Kluwer.

Spiva, L., Hart, P. L., Patrick, S., Waggoner, J., Jackson, C., & Threat, J. L. (2017). Effectiveness of an evidence-based practice nurse mentor training. *Worldviews on Evidence-Based Nursing, 14*(3), 183–191.

Strauss, S., Tetroe, J., & Graham, I. (2009). *Knowledge translation in health care.* Blackwell Publishing Ltd.

PEACE MODEL

P | **PROBLEM IDENTIFICATION**
Formulate the clinical question (**PICO**):
- **P** | Patient Population
- **I** | Intervention
- **C** | Comparison of Intervention
- **O** | Outcome

E | **EVIDENCE REVIEW**
Review evidence relevant to your clinical question by searching databases.

A | **APPRAISE EVIDENCE**
Appraise the evidence that appears highest in the hierarchy of scientific evidence for its quality and applicability to practice.

C | **CHANGE PRACTICE OR CONDUCT RESEARCH**
If evidence is sufficient, embark on improvement project to address practice change.
If evidence is insufficient to warrant practice change, conduct research.

E | **EVALUATE AND DISSEMINATE FINDINGS**
Evaluate the impact of the implemented practice change and research results.
Disseminate findings through publication, oral, and poster presentations.

10

PRACTICE EXEMPLARS

–Mary Rose Papciak, MPA, BSN, RN, NEA-BC

KEYWORDS | PHRASES
evidence-based practice (EBP), utilization framework, nurse resident,
clinical questions, PICO, exemplar projects, appraisal, dissemination,
quality improvement, research

CHAPTER OBJECTIVES

After studying this chapter, learners will be able to:

1. Delineate components of the NYP PEACE model and describe the process from problem identification to dissemination of findings.

2. Provide exemplars of evidence-based practice (EBP) and research that illustrate utilization of the NYP PEACE model through a five-step process.

3. Develop an EBP project using the NYP PEACE model.

Introduction

This chapter provides exemplars of evidence-based practice (EBP) projects and research at NewYork-Presbyterian (NYP) Hospital that illustrate utilization of the NYP PEACE model. Each exemplar is used to demonstrate clinical nurse-driven practice change or the conduct of research through successful application of the PEACE model. We describe the five-step process from problem identification through dissemination and evaluation of findings in each practice example.

As nurses, it is important to think critically and apply your knowledge to drive improved patient care and outcomes through EBP and research. EBP may seem challenging at first; however, when you know and understand how to apply the PEACE model, you will be able to follow the simple process to complete an EBP project and make an impact in changing practice. Through the examples shared in this chapter, you are provided with a guide to create your own EBP project leading to implementation of a practice change or dissemination of new knowledge through the conduct of research.

The PEACE model guides clinical nurses to identify and use available resources for obtaining scholarly evidence, research, and best practices in improving care of patients. It is a model to facilitate EBP review and the conduct and utilization of research. EBP and research projects start with identification of a problem, followed by formulation of a PICO question. Next steps include evidence review and appraisal, followed by changing practice or conducting research. For those clinical questions posed without sufficient evidence in the literature, nurses use the PEACE model to conduct research. Evaluation of an implemented practice change and dissemination of research findings are important final steps in the process.

In this chapter we use each exemplar to demonstrate the step-by-step process inherent in the PEACE model.

Step 1 | **P**EACE: Problem identification

Step 2 | P**E**ACE: Evidence review

Step 3 | PE**A**CE: Appraise the evidence

Step 4 | PEA**C**E: Conduct research or change practice

Step 5 | PEAC**E**: Evaluation and dissemination of findings

Exemplar 1
Delaying the Newborn Bath: A Nurse Residency Program Practice Change

–Mary Rose Papciak, MPA, BSN, RN, NEA-BC

The EBP project "Delaying the Newborn Bath" demonstrates our first example of a practice change implemented by using the PEACE model.

Four new graduate nurse residents developed this EBP project during their first year of practice. Throughout participation in the Nurse Residency Program (NRP), they worked together as a team to identify a problem relevant to their practice as mother/baby registered nurses (key stakeholders), conduct a literature review, and appraise the evidence. As a team, the nurse residents evaluated the current practice at NYP on the mother/baby unit and recommended a nursing practice change based on the evidence review.

For the purposes of the NRP, the new graduate nurses completed the first three steps of PEACE—problem identification, evidence review, and appraise evidence. Based upon their literature review, they recognized a clinical need to implement a practice change. Therefore, the team of nurse residents went further with their work to include the "C" and "E" steps of the model.

Exemplar 1 focuses on the clinical topic of delayed bathing of newborns delivered at or greater than 35 weeks gestation to improve patient outcomes.

Step 1 | PEACE
Problem Identification

Nurse residents reported a rise in parent requests to delay their newborns' bath, ranging from the initial hours of life to days after birth. Delayed bathing is a practice supported by various organizations, such as the World Health Organization and the American Academy of Pediatrics (Lund, 2016). Newborns are more susceptible to hypothermia than adults due to the increased surface area of an infant. Positive outcomes of this practice include increased parental bonding time with baby, increased breastfeeding rates, improved thermoregulation, and less incidence of hypoglycemia. As mother/baby nurses, the team of new graduate nurses were determined to provide the highest-quality, safest patient care for their patients, while also improving the patient experience. The purpose of this evidence-based project was to evaluate the effectiveness of delaying the newborn bath and to implement innovative ideas based on the evidence, keeping in line with the hospital's policy to provide quality, patient-centered care based on best practice.

Current nursing practices include using soap and water to bathe stable newborns under the radiant warmer upon admission. The nurse residents' goal was to engage key stakeholders in understanding the supporting evidence to their proposed practice change: delayed bathing.

The clinical question investigated was:

Among newborns delivered at or greater than 35 weeks gestation, admitted to the NYP Weill Cornell Medical Center well-baby nursery, does delaying the newborn's bath 12–24 hours after birth, compared to 2–4 hours, result in improved temperature regulation, blood glucose levels, and overall transition to the extra-uterine environment?

Step 2 | PEACE
Evidence Review

The team conducted a literature review using the NYP library resources available (PubMed). Inclusion criteria included articles published within the last five years and focused on the newborn population. The studies showed delayed bathing had a positive impact on breastfeeding rates, neonatal hypoglycemia, and thermoregulation of preterm infants. Evidence supporting this practice change aligns with the hospital's goal of becoming a baby-friendly organization. Nurse residents also summarized the evidence to support their clinical question.

Step 3 | PEACE
Appraise Evidence

After the strengths and limitations of the studies were reviewed, the Critical Appraisal Skills Programme (CASP) checklist was used to assess the quality of the studies. Strengths of the articles appraised included similar patient populations and transferability of findings to clinical settings. One article involved was a randomized controlled trial, which collected data pre- and post-bathing to monitor thermoregulation (Loring et al., 2012). Limitations included limited sample sizes based upon gestational age and high risk of hypoglycemia.

Step 4 | PEACE
Change Practice
(Recommendations and Next Steps)

After reviewing the literature, current practice, and patient preferences, the nurse residents recommended delaying the newborn bath at least 12 hours post-delivery (Preer et al., 2013). New graduate nurse residents also endorsed continued education to both patients and nurses on the benefits of skin-to-skin contact—which is supported by the delayed bath—thereby lessening maternal infant separation and further improving thermoregulation. By discussing this practice change with the nursing leadership team (key stakeholders), a plan for the pilot implementation was considered and launched on the postpartum unit. Both clinical nurses and parents were educated on the benefits of delayed bathing to further promote compliance.

Step 5 | PEAC**E**
Evaluation and Dissemination of Findings

Next up for the team was dissemination of findings with their colleagues in nursing, unit leadership, and medical providers, as well as proposing implementation of the delayed bath on the postpartum nursing unit. Additionally, the team encouraged and supported the new practice change to improve patient outcomes.

An evaluation of benefits was conducted on the postpartum unit, and practice change was later expanded to a second unit as a result of the positive outcomes.

Discussion: This project was presented to the nursing leadership team during the NRP graduation celebration in the form of a poster presentation. It was further shared at the unit level and presented to the nursing practice council for policy revision and update. Nurse residents received support from the medical provider team during implementation as well, which contributed to their success. Feedback has been positive since implementation, and the practice has received interest at various NYP sites across the enterprise. This new knowledge has been nationally disseminated at the Vizient/AACN Nurse Residency Program™ conference.

Acknowledgment: The authors want to recognize the clinical nurses and nurse leaders at NYP Hospital who participated in the development of this exemplar—specifically, Tammy Leung, BSN, RN; Veronica Pasha, BSN, RN; Stephanie Savage, BSN, RN; and Bethany Saduddin-Singh, BSN, RN.

Exemplar 2
Post-Stroke Depression: Nursing Knowledge and Practice Implications

–Jason R. Johnson, BSN, RN, SCRN, Clinical Nurse I, Cardiothoracic ICU

Step 1 | **P**EACE
Problem Identification

Stroke is the fifth leading cause of death in the United States and one of the major causes of physical disability. Ischemic and hemorrhagic strokes can lead to numerous complications, including motor weakness, aphasia, dysphagia, visual disturbances, seizures, and pneumonia. Disability related to stroke is most often characterized by functional disability, though impaired cognition (e.g., impairment of memory, attention, and executive functioning) can also be found.

Neurological patients in general, and stroke patients in particular, often experience psychiatric distress, such as euphoria, disinhibition, and helplessness. However, the most common form of emotional upset in the stroke patient is depression. Post-stroke depression can affect anywhere from 30% to 50% of stroke patients, with the risk highest immediately after the stroke event, up to one-year post-stroke. Post-stroke depression can result in reduced participation in rehabilitation activities, leading to decreased functional and cognitive recovery.

Step 2 | PEACE
Evidence Review

A literature review was conducted primarily utilizing the Cumulative Index to Nursing and Allied Health Literature (CINAHL) database. Inclusion criteria included articles specifically on nursing implication of post-stroke depression, post-stroke depression epidemiology and pathophysiology, and post-stroke depression screening. Search results were limited to articles published in the last five years.

Step 3 | PEACE
Appraise Evidence

The literature supports the use of early screening protocols for depression in stroke patients. The existing literature strongly supports the use of brief screening tools by clinical nurses to utilize in screening for post-stroke depression, and there is evidence of the value of assessing baseline nursing knowledge and perceptions related to depression in cardiac patients. However, few studies address the underlying issue of baseline knowledge level of clinical nurses on post-stroke depression as a major stroke complication, as well as the ability to screen for it early in the clinical course. If nurses are not aware of depression as a stroke complication, they cannot appropriately screen stroke patients for it.

The aim of the study was to determine the baseline knowledge level and beliefs of clinical nurses on a high-acuity neurosurgery stepdown unit related to post-stroke depression, as well as to determine whether a brief educational intervention can increase the knowledge level of nurses to have the foundation to intervene early to prevent further complications.

Step 4 | PEACE
Conduct Research

This study was a pretest-posttest pilot study on a 36-bed neurosurgery stepdown unit. At the time of study completion, there were 52 registered nurses employed on the unit. Staff primarily hold a bachelor of science in nursing, two are stroke certified registered nurses, two are neuroscience certified registered nurses, and two are certified in medical-surgical nursing. One nurse also is designated a clinical nurse III (CN III), the highest level on the clinical ladder advancement program for clinical nurses at the bedside at this institution. The unit is also led by a master's-prepared RN, the patient care director. Participants for this study were drawn solely from clinical bedside nurses on the neurosurgery stepdown unit.

Participants completed the Post-Stroke Depression Knowledge and Attitudes Survey (PSD-KAS), a 32-item, author-designed survey that assesses knowledge and attitudes related to depression in general and post-stroke depression in particular. Survey items were rated on a Likert scale, ranging from strongly disagree (1 out of 5) to strongly agree (5 out of 5).

Following the pre-survey phase of the study, participants received an educational intervention focused on increasing basic clinical knowledge related to post-stroke depression. This educational intervention was given in small groups throughout clinical shifts of the participants. The intervention consisted of a brief, 15-minute in-service on the basics of post-stroke depression, common etiologies, epidemiology, clinical bedside nurse screening, and treatment strategies.

After the intervention phase of the study was complete, post-surveys were distributed to study participants. The post-survey consisted of the PSD-KAS, with two additional questions querying whether the participant completed the pre-survey or the educational intervention.

Step 5 | PEACE
Evaluation and Dissemination of Findings

Forty-six of 52 nurses completed the pre-survey, an 88.46% response rate; 39 of 52 nurses completed the post-survey, a 75% response rate. Mean score on pre-survey was 91.61 (SD: 4.21) out of 160, indicating slightly low (less than average) knowledge related to depression in general and post-stroke depression in particular. Mean score on the post-survey was 136.92 (SD: 6.98) out of 160, indicating high (greater than average) knowledge related to depression in general and post-stroke depression in particular.

Knowledge related to this study has been disseminated at local and national nursing conferences, including the American Association of Neuroscience Nurses' (AANN) annual educational meeting, the AANN Advances in Stroke Care Conference, and the Academy of Medical-Surgical Nurses' annual conference. The aim of this work is publication in a peer-reviewed journal.

Discussion: This project was presented in the NRP as a poster presentation and serves as an exemplar for new nurse residents. After completing the NRP, Jason Johnson, BSN, RN, SCRN participated in the NYP Academic Practice Research Fellowship and submitted his work for publication in the *Journal of Neuroscience Nursing* in September 2019. Mr. Johnson completed requested revisions in 2019 and re-submitted for publication in January 2020. He is awaiting a response on publication.

Acknowledgment: Jason R. Johnson, BSN, RN, SCRN, Clinical Nurse I, Cardiothoracic ICU

Exemplar 3
Tai Chi to Reduce Falls in the Geriatric Population

–Avis Russ, MBA, MS, BSN, RN, NE-BC
–Elza Rosen, BSN, BS, RN
–Sarah Otto, BSN, RN

Elza Rosen, BSN, BS, RN, and Sarah Otto, BSN, RN, participated in the NYP NRP as new graduate clinical nurses. As part of the NRP, Rosen and Otto collaborated on an EBP project on falls risk due to the prevalence of falls and fall risks among the geriatric population. The fall prevention protocol at the time included the use of chair alarms, bed pad alarms, patient fall and injury prevention education, physical therapy evaluations, and assistive devices such as wheelchairs and walkers, night lights, and high fall risk alerts (yellow wrist band and yellow non-skid socks) and yoga.

Step 1 | PEACE
Problem Identification

Rosen and Otto were concerned that patients continued to fall despite implementation of the current fall prevention protocol. The clinical question investigated was:

"Does implementing the practice of tai chi twice per week in 15-minute seg-ments in adults 65 years and older reduce the occurrence of falls compared to those who do not practice tai chi?"

Step 2 | PEACE
Evidence Review

Rosen and Otto conducted a literature search to collect evidence and best practices about fall reduction interventions that were not being included in the current fall prevention protocol. Evidence revealed that the use of tai chi reduced the inci-dence of falls in the 65 years of age and older population. At NYPH/Westchester Behavioral Health Center (WBHC), the current fall prevention protocol at that time consisted of chair alarms, bed pad alarms, patient fall and injury prevention education, physical therapy evaluations, assistive devices (such as wheelchairs and walkers), night lights, high fall risk alerts (such as yellow wrist bands and yellow nonskid socks), and yoga. As part of their search for the best evidence, the clinical nurses found that incorporating tai chi on a daily basis for 10 minutes reduced the incidence of falls in the 65 years of age and older population (Li et al., 2016). Tai chi was found to be an evidence-based fall reduction intervention that answered their clinical question.

Step 3 | PEACE
Appraise Evidence

Rosen and Otto reviewed articles related to fall prevention protocols in the geriatric population of patients. Articles on the use of tai chi were critiqued using the CASP tool. Literature reviewed was determined to be of good quality, and the nurses recommended a new practice intervention to support fall reduction.

Step 4 | PEACE
Change Practice

Based on the findings, the clinical nurses were interested in making a proposal to revise the current fall prevention protocol by adding the use of tai chi as a new falls prevention intervention to improve care with the goal of reducing falls among the geriatric population. Tai chi was incorporated into the activity schedule for patients meeting certain criteria on a geriatric psychiatry unit at NYPH/WBHC.

Rosen moved forward with her proposal to revise the existing fall prevention protocol by adding a supervised tai chi group twice a week that would be taught by the geriatric unit nurses in 15-minute segments. The goal was revised for the existing practice to add tai chi, an evidence-based intervention that was shown to be effective in decreasing fall incidences, increasing gait stability, and reducing fear of falling within the geriatric population.

Step 5 | PEAC**E**
Evaluation and Dissemination of Findings

The NRP evidence-based project of Rosen and Otto culminated in a poster presentation at the NRP graduation on March 8, 2017. Their poster presented the next steps of their project to clinical nurses and the leadership team. They proposed that the current fall prevention protocol be revised by adding a supervised tai chi group taught by nurses twice a week in 15-minute segments, with the goal of improving care by reducing fall incidences, increasing gait stability, and reducing fear of falling among the geriatric population.

Following dissemination of findings through a poster presentation, Rosen received advisement to continue implementation of the EBP project by members of NYPH/WBHC's New Knowledge, Innovations, and Improvements (NK) team (key stakeholders). The NK team, composed of nurses at all levels, is critical to assisting nurses with research, EBP, and quality projects.

Evaluation is an important step when implementing a practice change. In September 2017, a proposal to revise the existing geriatric unit fall prevention protocol was presented to the Psychiatric Nurse Practice Council. It was discussed that evidence-based findings support the use of tai chi in reducing falls and improving care. This revision to existing nursing practice as a pilot program was approved by the Psychiatric Nurse Practice Council at NYPH/WBHC.

Rosen coordinated the plan for the revision of the existing geriatric unit fall prevention protocol with her nurse manager. Rosen was advised to involve the interprofessional team, which would offer her additional support with sustaining the change. She received approval from the team to incorporate tai chi into the patient schedules and assistance from the medical group to offer medical clearance, which could be provided by advanced practice registered nurses. Rosen sought assistance from physical therapists to incorporate readiness for tai chi as part of their initial admission assessments. To facilitate the tai chi groups, she accessed available resources to secure videos, which she located at public libraries.

Rosen introduced the practice revision involving the fall prevention protocol and the introduction of tai chi to her peers at the September Unit Practice Council (UPC) meeting. At this meeting, she suggested a once-weekly intervention; however, she later decided to implement the tai chi group twice a week, which was recommended as part of the original proposal. During the UPC meeting, she showed excerpts from several tai chi videos to her peers to obtain their buy-in for the practice change and to have them weigh in on the choice of a video. The members chose a video titled "Fu Style: Healing Exercise—The Power to Heal Yourself Sitting Tai Chi" due to the video's slow and clear instructions, which included breathing exercises that allowed for timed breaks. Rosen also developed a patient education handout with explanations and benefits about tai chi.

The nurses used the tai chi patient education handout as a teaching tool to educate the patients about tai chi prior to their voluntary participation. Rosen educated the unit nurses before the first group on where the video would be stored to ensure the groups were conducted twice weekly. Nurses were prepared for the group by watching a portion of the videos and reviewing the handout prior to the first group.

In early October 2017, the first tai chi group was conducted, with the group planned for Sundays and Mondays thereafter. Rosen facilitated the first tai chi group and supervised the patients in the dayroom as the video played. Ten patients participated, and at the end of the group, the patients reported feeling relaxed and focused and commented that they wanted this group to become a part of the routine unit schedule. Tai chi groups have continued to be implemented twice weekly.

Discussion: December 2017 data showed a reduction in patient falls on the inpatient geriatric unit, and reports of improved care continue to be evaluated. In the spring of 2017, Rosen and Otto participated in an annual poster showcase at NYPH/WBHC to further disseminate this new knowledge and practice change.

Acknowledgment: The authors want to recognize the clinical nurses and nurse leaders at NYP Hospital who participated in the development of this exemplar.

Exemplar 4
Video-Based Education to Reduce Distress and Improve Understanding Among Pediatric MRI Patients

–Dan Hogan, MSN, RN, CCRN

This exemplar describes a pilot randomized controlled trial conducted in a large, urban academic children's hospital. This example will walk you through the steps a clinical nurse took using the PEACE model that led him to the conduct of research.

Step 1 | PEACE
Problem Identification

Magnetic Resonance Imaging (MRI) exams can cause distress, such as fear and anxiety, especially in the pediatric population (Koller & Goldman, 2012). Because of this distress and the need to get high-quality studies, pediatric patients often require sedation or anesthesia. The use of anesthesia comes with increased risks to patient safety, increased cost, and increased time at visit (Barnea-Gorlaly et al., 2014). One of the key strategies used to reduce distress in patients undergoing a medical procedure is providing age-appropriate education to patients and their caretakers. When a staff member's school-age niece was scheduled for an MRI, she asked her aunt what an MRI was and what she should expect. Her aunt, a nurse practitioner (NP) in the Pediatric Diagnostic and Interventional Radiology Department, attempted to show her a video but had difficulty finding a suitable video online. When the NP and charge nurse (CN) of the unit investigated current education available on their own unit, they found that pediatric patients who were about to undergo an MRI exam received varying degrees of education prior to the exam. The content and length of education provided was mainly dependent on the experience, knowledge base, and comfort level of the MRI staff, as well as the time they had available to provide education and answer any questions from the patients or their caretakers.

The NP and CN met with the nurse manager of the unit to discuss their findings and see if there was a way to standardize the education given to the patients and their caretakers. Because of the lack of suitable videos available online, the perceived engagement level of the MRI staff, and the generally preferred learning style of the targeted population, the team decided that an educational video would be the best tool. Subsequently, a seven-minute educational video was developed by an interprofessional healthcare team that included nurses, MRI technologists, and a child life specialist. The clinical question investigated was:

What is the impact of an educational video on minimizing distress among pediatric patients that are about to undergo an MRI exam?

Step 2 | PEACE
Evidence Review

The research team conducted a literature review using the library resources available. Inclusion criteria were articles published within the past five years and focused on tools used to decrease distress such as anxiety, pain, and nervousness in pediatric patients who were about to undergo an exam or medical procedure. Although several studies focused on the use of distraction tools to decrease distress for procedures such as blood lab draws (phlebotomy) and peripheral intravenous line insertions, there were a limited number of studies involving MRI. Due to the limited number of studies, the team altered the initial inclusion criteria to include articles published within the past 10 years. Because increasing the inclusion criteria did not yield a relatively large increase in results, the team decided to conduct a randomized controlled study comparing distress levels of pediatric patients about to undergo an MRI with usual standard of care versus those who received the video-based education (Hogan et al., 2018).

Step 3 | PEACE
Appraise Evidence

After reviewing the evidence by the research team, strengths and weaknesses were listed to assess the quality of the studies. Strengths of the articles appraised included similar patient populations in terms of age, distress, and disposition to preprocedure or test. Limitations included limited sample sizes, use of multimodal approaches, and a single-modal approach that did not include video-based education.

Step 4 | PEACE
Conduct Research & Change Practice

Based on insufficient evidence in the literature, the team moved forward with conducting research. A randomized controlled study was done, which led to recommendation of a practice change. After reviewing the results of the randomized controlled study, the nurse manager and charge nurse recommended standardizing patient education utilizing the video-based education tool. The MRI team received education regarding the new practice and support from nursing leadership during implementation. Feedback was positive during implementation, and the practice has received interest in other departments within the institution where the study was conducted.

This education tool was available to patients and their caretakers via a web link that was provided to them during a preprocedure phone call. For those caretakers who did not have access to the internet or did not have the chance to review the video prior to their appointment, an opportunity to view the video was made available to them during the wait time of their scheduled visit. Upon arrival to their appointment, the MRI nurse or technician introduced themselves and gave the caretakers the pre-MRI screening form. At this time, an inquiry was made on whether the patient/caretaker had watched the video. If the patient/caretaker denied having watched the video, a mobile tablet with the video was provided in a quiet waiting area to allow viewing of the educational material prior to the procedure.

Step 5 | PEAC**E**
Evaluation and Dissemination of Findings

The team shared their research findings with their colleagues in nursing, unit leadership, and medical providers, as well as proposed implementation of the video-based education prior to the MRI exam. The team encouraged and supported the new practice change to improve patient experience and patient outcomes.

This research study was published in the *Journal of Pediatric Nursing* (Hogan et al., 2018).

Discussion: This project was presented to participants of the Nursing Research Symposium "Nurses Advancing Science and Improving Patient Care" at NYP Hospital (November 2016) as a poster presentation. The charge nurse who first noted the varying degrees of education provided to patients and their caretakers prior to an MRI was invited and spoke at several research committees and was part of a nurse panel titled "Clinical Research in Action: Lessons Learned." The research was also presented in the form of a poster at the Morgan Stanley Children's Hospital's "Parade of Posters" during Nursing Week of 2017.

Acknowledgment: The authors want to recognize the MRI staff and nurse leaders at NYP Hospital who supported the making of the video as well as the randomized controlled study that resulted from this project. Specifically, Mely Chua, MPH, RN; Heidi Jerome, MD; and Steve Barrena, RN.

Exemplar 5
Addressing the Barriers of Certification Through the Certification Ambassador Program

–Warly Remegio, DNP, RN, NPD-BC, CCRN-CSC

NYP Department of Nursing's vision is to be one of the nation's leaders in nursing practice, quality, safety, outcomes, nursing research, education, and service excellence. To support this vision, one of the goals is to employ a multitude of strategies, including the validation of the expertise and continued competency of nurses through national board certification. The organization aims to promote and sustain a culture of certification, which plays a significant role in leveraging nursing professional competence, empowerment, and job satisfaction and in improving patient care outcomes (Boyle et al., 2014; Coelho, 2020; Conley, 2019; Perlstein et al., 2014).

This recently implemented evidence-based and performance improvement project utilized the PEACE model with the goal of increasing certification across the organization. This collaborative project focuses on multimodal approaches to address the barriers to certification using the Certification Ambassador Program.

Step 1 | PEACE
Problem Identification

In December 2017, NYP Lower Manhattan Hospital (LMH) had overall certification rates of 22%. In 2018, the goal was to increase the certification rate by 2%. With this goal, the Department of Nursing formed a Certification Steering Committee to address the barriers to certification and to assist the organization in increasing its certification rate. The steering committee was composed of Warly Remegio, DNP, RN, NPD-BC, CCRN-CSC, Program Director for Nursing Professional Development; Reynaldo Rivera, DNP, RN, NEA-BC, FAAN, Director of Nursing for Nursing Research and Innovation; Alexandra Shelley, MS, RN-BC, FNP-BC, Clinical Program Coordinator (clinical nurse at the time); Lisandra Torres, MSN, RNC-OB, C-EFM, Labor and Delivery Patient Care Director (PCD); Beth Taubkin, MS, RN, CPAN, Nurse Educator; and Annalisse Mahon, MSN, RN, Operating Room PCD. The committee conducted a survey to clinical nurses in all the clinical units on their perceived barriers and facilitators to obtaining certification. There were more than 200 responses to the survey from various clinical areas. Figures 10.1 and 10.2 include the summary of the results.

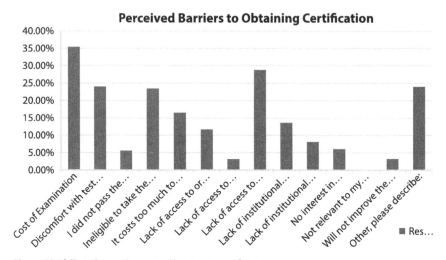

Figure 10.1 | Clinical nurses' perceived barriers to certification.

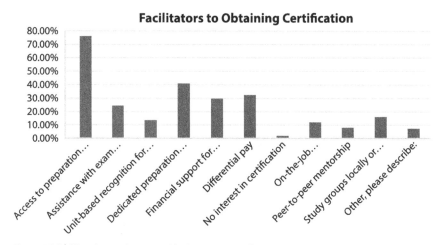

Figure 10.2 | Clinical nurses' perceived facilitators to certification.

Step 2 | PEACE
Evidence Review

Based on the feedback from the clinical nurses, the certification steering committee gathered and reviewed the most recent literature addressing the barriers to certification. The team had utilized nursing library resources like PubMed, CINAHL, EBSCO, and other nursing/healthcare databases in searching for certification programs and initiatives addressing the barriers to obtaining certification. The key terms used included *nursing certification, specialty certification initiatives, certification barriers*, and *facilitators*. This search was limited to five years in acute care settings.

Step 3 | PEACE
Appraise Evidence

The steering committee appraised the evidence and took into consideration the outcomes and settings of those studies. Some of the key interventions noted include:

- Providing robust resources for certification within the organization
- Conducting formal review sessions
- Providing certification incentives
- Recognition and rewards
- Conducting informal small group review sessions
- Providing education on the available certification resources
- Leadership and peer-to-peer support

These noted interventions are congruent to the survey results taken by the nurses regarding the facilitators to obtaining certification. With this, the committee developed an innovative program that could bundle evidence-based interventions through the implementation of a Certification Ambassador Program (CAP).

Step 4 | PEA**C**E
Change Practice

The CAP aims to empower nationally board-certified clinical nurses as active ambassadors in fostering a culture of professional excellence through certification of nurses throughout the organization. Certified registered nurses with interest in promoting certification achievement were invited to join a certification ambassador retreat, which was held in October 2018. The nurses were trained as ambassadors, and resources for certification were provided, based on a curriculum developed by the steering committee. The ambassadors also discussed how to address the barriers from the survey and from the literature, which included lack of access to preparations courses, lack of support, lack of rewards and recognition, and discomfort with tests (Perlstein et al., 2014). The CAP was formally implemented later in October with engaged ambassadors from various clinical areas. The Certification Ambassador Champions began promoting unit nurse certification, educating colleagues on the importance of obtaining certification and the resources available for certification, assisting others in obtaining certification through peer-to-peer support, assisting with coordinating unit-based study groups, and answering questions about certification eligibility and other NYP-LMH certification resources. Their role included collaborating with the educators and unit PCDs to champion certification as well as finding ways to recognize and celebrate those who become certified in their respective units. Additionally, the certification steering committee worked collaboratively with Nursing Professional Development in offering various certification review sessions throughout the year within the organization. Clinical nurses were encouraged and supported to attend those classes. The steering committee also worked with the Recruitment, Recognition, and Retention (R3) Committee in holding Certification Day Recognition and celebration events to honor the newly certified nurses, including all those certified nurses who gained their certification in the previous years. During the 2019 ceremony, the R3 Committee recognized nearly 35 newly certified nurses.

Step 5 | PEAC**E**
Evaluation and Dissemination of Findings

This innovative role development strategy was instrumental in cultivating a culture of certification, engagement, and professional excellence throughout the organization.

At the end of 2018, the organization had achieved 35% certification rate, a 4% increase from the previous year. To date, the organization has achieved 40%, with more clinical nurses aspiring to become certified this year. These results are included in Figure 10.3.

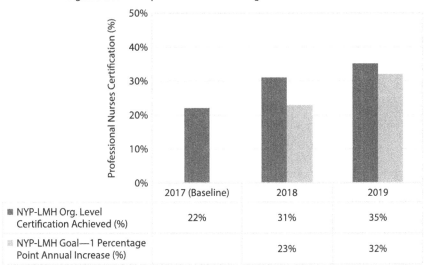

NYP-LMH Organizational Level Certification Rate (%) 2017–2019
Targeted Goal for Improvement—1 Percentage Point Annual Increase

	2017 (Baseline)	2018	2019
NYP-LMH Org. Level Certification Achieved (%)	22%	31%	35%
NYP-LMH Goal—1 Percentage Point Annual Increase (%)		23%	32%

Figure 10.3 | NYP-LMH organization level of certification rate (%) 2017–2019.

Discussion: Eliciting clinical nurses' feedback is key in creating innovative and relevant strategies to address the barriers to obtaining certification. The ongoing partnership and collaboration between nurse educators, nurse leaders, and clinical nurses strengthens the culture of engagement and commitment to certification. The notable outcome on this initiative made it highly recommended to other NYP campuses to achieve an enterprise-wide increase in certification. Empowering the ambassadors and the newly certified clinical nurses to become leaders and mentors of certification reaffirms our commitment to professional excellence and to excellent nursing and patient care outcomes.

Acknowledgment: Warly Remegio, DNP, RN, NPD-BC, CCRN-CSC; Reynaldo R. Rivera, DNP, RN, NEA-BC, FAAN; Eileen Cater, PhD, RN; and the LMH Certification Steering Committee.

Summary

This chapter describes how clinical nurses identified best practices through supporting evidence to change practice or lack thereof, resulting in the need to conduct research. We hope you find that the PEACE model five-step process is simple and easy to use. The PEACE model can be your guide for successful EBP projects as well as research, and we encourage you to use this framework to advance nursing science. It is our goal that through sharing these exemplars, you will be confident to break through existing barriers and engage in EBP and research.

Review Questions

1. The integration of best practices, patient preferences, and clinician expertise into patient care is called what?

   Answer: Evidence-based practice

2. What is the first step in the utilization of the PEACE model, and what tool may help you further define your clinical question?

   Answer: Problem identification, PICO process

3. If you ask a clinical question and are unable to find sufficient evidence in the literature, what is your next step?

   Answer: Conduct research

4. When utilizing the PEACE model, what are two important final steps after implementing a practice change?

   Answer: Evaluation of the practice change and dissemination of findings

5. What clinical question do you have, and why is it important to nursing practice? Write your own PICO question to start using the PEACE model.

   Answer: Open ended question. Readers will create a PICO question and write a response based on their own clinical experience or specialty topic of interest that may lead to an EBP project.

References

Barnea-Goraly, N., Weinzimer, S. A., Ruedy, K. J., Mauras, N., Beck, R. W., Marzelli, M. J., Mazaika, P. K., Aye, T., White, N. H., Tsalikian, E., Fox, L., Kollman, C., Cheng, P., Reiss, A. L., & Diabetes Research in Children Network (DirecNet). (2014). High success rates of sedation-free brain MRI scanning in young children using simple subject preparation protocols with and without a commercial mock scanner—the Diabetes Research in Children Network (DirecNet) experience. *Pediatric Radiology, 44*(2), 181–186. https://doi.org/10.1007/s00247-013-2798-7

Boyle, D. K., Cramer, E., Potter, C., Gatua, M. W., & Stobinski, J. X. (2014). The relationship between direct-care RN specialty certification and surgical patient outcomes. *AORN Journal, 100*(5), 511–528. https://doi.org/10.1016/j.aorn.2014.04.018

Coelho, P. (2020). Relationship between nurse certification and clinical patient outcomes: A systematic literature review. *Journal of Nursing Care Quality, 35*(1), E1–E5. https://doi.org/10.1097/NCQ.0000000000000397

Conley, P. (2019). Certified and advanced degree critical care nurses improve patient outcomes. *Dimensions of Critical Care Nursing, 38*(2), 108–112.

Hogan, D., DiMartino, T., Liu, J., Mastro, K. A., Larson, E., & Carter, E. (2018). Video-based education to reduce distress and improve understanding among pediatric MRI patients: A randomized controlled study. *Journal of Pediatric Nursing, 41*, 48–53. https://doi.org/10.1016/j.pedn.2018.01.005

Koller, D., & Goldman, R. D. (2012). Distraction techniques for children undergoing procedures: A critical review of pediatric research. *Journal of Pediatric Nursing, 27*(6), 652–681. https://doi.org/10.1016/j.pedn.2011.08.001

Li, F., Harmer, P., & Fitzgerald, K. (2016). Implementing an evidence-based fall prevention intervention in community senior centers. *American Journal of Public Health, 106*(11), 2026–2031. https://doi.org/10.2105/AJPH.2016.303386

Loring, C., Gregory, K., Gargan, B., LeBlanc, V., Lundgren, D., Reilly, J., Stobo, K., Walker, C., & Zaya, C. (2012). Tub bathing improves thermoregulation of the late preterm infant. *Journal of Obstetric, Gynecologic, and Neonatal Nursing, 41*(2), 171–179. https://doi.org/10.1111/j.1552-6909.2011.01332.x

Lund, C. (2016). Bathing and beyond: Current bathing controversies for newborn infants. *Advances in Neonatal Care, 16*, S13–S20. https://doi.org/10.1097/ANC.0000000000000336

Perlstein, L., Hoffmann, R. L., Lindberg, J., & Petras, D. (2014). Addressing barriers to achieving nursing certification: Development of a certification achievement program on a medical-surgical unit. *Journal for Nurses in Professional Development, 30*(6), 309–315. https://doi.org/10.1097/NND.0000000000000115

Preer, G., Pisegna, J. M., Cook, J. T., Henri, A. M., & Philipp, B. L. (2013). Delaying the bath and in-hospital breastfeeding rates. *Breastfeeding Medicine, 8*(6), 485–490. https://doi.org/10.1089/bfm.2012.0158

INDEX

NOTE: Page reference noted with a *t* are tables; page references noted with an *f* are figures

I

J–K

L